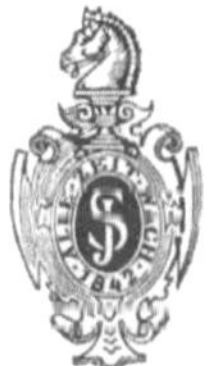

Recent Results in Cancer Research

Fortschritte der Krebsforschung

Progrès dans les recherches sur le cancer

18

Edited by

V. G. Allfrey, New York · M. Allgöwer, Basel · K. H. Bauer, Heidelberg · I. Berenblum, Rehovoth · F. Bergel, Jersey, C. I. · J. Bernard, Paris · W. Bernhard, Villejuif N. N. Blokhin, Moskva · H. E. Bock, Tübingen · P. Bucalossi, Milano · A. V. Chaklin, Moskva · M. Chorazy, Gliwice · G. J. Cunningham, London · W. Dameshek, Boston M. Dargent, Lyon · G. Della Porta, Milano · P. Denoix, Villejuif · R. Dulbecco, La Jolla · H. Eagle, New York · E. Eker, Oslo · P. Grabar, Paris · H. Hamperl, Bonn R. J. C. Harris, London · E. Hecker, Heidelbreg · R. Herbeuval, Nancy · J. Higginson, Lyon · W. C. Hueper, Fort Myers, Florida · H. Isliker, Lausanne · D. A. Karnofsky, New York · J. Kieler, København · G. Klein, Stockholm · H. Koprowski, Philadelphia · L. G. Koss, New York · G. Martz, Zürich · G. Mathé, Villejuif · O. Mühlbock, Amsterdam · W. Nakahara, Tokyo · G. T. Pack, New York · V. R. Potter, Madison · A. B. Sabin, Cincinnati · L. Sachs, Rehovoth · E. A. Saxén, Helsinki W. Szybulski, Madison · H. Tagnon, Bruxelles · R. M. Taylor, Toronto · A. Tissières, Genève · E. Uehlinger, Zürich · R. W. Wissler, Chicago · T. Yoshida, Tokyo

Editor in chief

P. Rentchnick, Genève

Springer-Verlag Berlin · Heidelberg · New York 1969

The Treatment of Hodgkin's Disease

By

Enrico Anglesio

With 30 Figures

Springer-Verlag Berlin · Heidelberg · New York 1969

*Professor Dr. Enrico Anglesio, Head of Department of Hormone-Chemotherapy,
Member effective of G.E.C.A. (Groupe Européen pour la Chimiothérapie
Anticancereuse), Institute of Oncology, Torino/Italy*

Sponsored by the Swiss League against Cancer

ISBN-13: 978-3-642-48268-7   e-ISBN-13: 978-3-642-48266-3
DOI: 10.1007/978-3-642-48266-3
Softcover reprint of the hardcover 1st edtion 1969

To *Margaret*
taking its place to support the others, . . .
With the drawing of this Love and the voice of this Calling

(T. S. Eliot — Four Quartets)

Preface

The discussion of some diseases is only occasionally enlivened by the emergence of new worthwhile facts. In the case of others, it would seem that, even if only a few years have passed, each new discussion wears the air of a revolution.

Hodgkin's disease, at least from the pathological standpoint, is not so extraordinarily fickle and certainly does not touch either of these two extremes of variability. But it is still a fertile field of study and presents its full share of innovations and practical results. This is perhaps due to the special position it occupies between tumours and inflammatory diseases, or possibly to a lucky series of coincidences; the truth is that events have been on the move for some years now in the case of this disease.

There can be no doubt that surprising progress has been made in connection with Hodgkin's disease, due, one feels, to close cooperation between several branches of medical science, each of which has had occasion to make new and useful contributions. This does not, however, hide the fact that certain important matters are still not clear, in particular the cause of the disease, its essential nature and, indeed, the best method for its treatment. Yet the success that has so far crowned the combined efforts of so many workers offers a shining example of the fruits to be gathered from close cooperation, and one which could well be extended to other fields. It is not too much to describe it as one of the success stories of modern medicine.

Torino, February 1968   ENRICO ANGLESIO

Contents

Chapter I

Historical Introduction

In a paper entitled "On some morbid appearances of the absorbent glands and spleen", written in 1832, THOMAS HODGKIN dealt with some forms of lymphoma, including (according to modern opinion) granuloma. The later history of the disease (Table 1), soon to bear his name, saw a number of important changes as similar morbid forms were hived off from his general description, a not uncommon process when opinions are divided and the number of cases is small.

Table 1. *History of Hodgkin's disease*

Year	Event
1832	1st description of lymph node disease by T. HODGKIN
1865	Name "Hodgkin's disease" proposed by WILKS
1897	PALTAUF's study of histological structure
1898	Description of tissue by STERNBERG
1902	Description of giant cells by DOROTHY REED
1903	1st radiotherapic management (SENN)
1904	Name "malignant granuloma" proposed by BENDA
1910	Discovery of FRAENKEL and MUCH granules in tissue
1911	Description of clinical course (ZIEGLER)
1913	Aetiology attributed to Corynebacterium (BUNTING and YATES)
1920	1st clinical classification (LONGCOPE et al.)
1939	GORDON's ultravirus experiments
1939	Aetiology attributed to Brucellae
1946	1st successful treatment with HN_2 (GOODMAN et al.)
1947	1st histological classification (JACKSON and PARKER)
1950	Stage classification of PETERS
1954	Discovery of delayed sensitivity (SCHIER)
1954	Accelerator X-ray beam treatment
1960	1st results of Vincaleucoblastine treatment
1962	Clinical classification of KAPLAN
1963	1st results of Methylhydrazine treatment
1963	2nd histological classification (LUKES)

Different trends in the treatment of Hodgkin's disease have their origins in its uncertain pathology and aetiology as well as in the advent of new forms of therapy. The discovery of X-rays in 1896 was followed by that of their effectiveness in certain blood and haematopoietic diseases. Successes were observed in the treatment of various forms of lymph node swelling, including Hodgkin's disease (1903).

At first, the variety of forms involved and the use of insufficient doses led to inconsistent result patterns, but with increased experience and technical improvements, culminating in the electron accelerators of to-day, success rates became higher.

For many years, the only medical alternative to radiotherapy was arsenic. This drug was used mainly as a complement in the treatment of anaemia during intervals in radiological therapy. Surgery was rarely resorted to.

The use of nitrogen mustard in the treatment of lymph node tumours and Hodgkin's disease began in 1946 (GOODMAN et al.) and opened a new road towards the treatment of diseases of the blood and lymphatic systems, including malignant tumours. New drugs, particularly those effective against radio-resistant and generalised forms, have contributed to the improvement of many patients.

Aetiopathogenetic theory was guided both by microscopical evidence and clinical course. As one or other of these factors prevailed, so there was a danger of Hodgkin's disease being confused with other lymph node abnormalities. The gradual build-up of pathological and clinical information, however, enabled KUNDRAT, TROUSSEAU, PALTAUF and STERNBERG to complete the work of differentiation. STERNBERG described the special tissue features of the disease and the giant cells bear his name.

The aetiology of the disease, however, is by no means clear. It was long thought to be a form, albeit weak, of tuberculosis. This view was supported by the finding of tubercular tissue and giant cells in the affected lymph nodes, by the presence of acid-fast granules (Much's granules) in tissue, by experimental evidence from the injection of guineapigs with glandular material, by the structure of the diseased tissue and by the febrile course. Bacterial or viral agents were sought and BUNTING and YATES (1913) isolated Corynebacterium Hodgkinii, the causative organism of Hodgkin-like but not identical lesions in monkeys. Brucellae were also suspected (PARSONS and POSTON, 1939; WISE and POSTON 1940; FORBUS et al., 1941) and the virus theory has received some attention in recent years following the experiments of GORDON (BOSTICK, 1958). This worker injected rabbit brain with Hodgkin lymphatic materials and induced fatal meningo-encephalitis. Material from these brains was found to contain a filtrable element including what have been described as primitive corpuscles. Others (MAGRASSI, BARBIERI) have shown, however, that the virus theory is not entirely convincing.

Although evidence of the precise agent is lacking, various data give life to the theory that the disease is the result of infection. These include: symptoms (e. g. fever), normal onset (in most cases, single site) in laterocervical lymph nodes, suggesting the pharyngotonsillar area as a focus or point of entry (ENNUYER et al., 1961), or, in other forms, onset in the intestine followed by metastasis to adjacent nodes. Over the last 20 years, however, increasing support has been given the view that the disease is of tumoral origin. Atypical mitoses have been observed in Sternberg cells and attention has been drawn to the complete destruction of surrounding lymphatic tissue and to the fact that the disease spreads to the remaining lymphatic apparatus, with infiltration of many organs and tissues. Successful radiotherapy and surgical excision of primary sites, coupled with the observation of frankly malignant tumoral forms (Hodgkin's sarcoma), have also lent weight to this theory.

The disease has also been attributed to a change in immunological status. This view has gained ground over the last 15 years since the studies of DUBIN and came into prominence with the first observations of T. B. anergy. Support for this view is also found in the behaviour patterns of the disease. Negative transfer of delayed sensitivity (SCHIER, 1954), skin-negative reactions to various chemical and bacterial allergens, coupled with delayed rejections of homografts, are signs that seem to fit in with the extensive destruction of lymphatic tissue. Lack of immune defence against infection seems also to be a typical feature of Hodgkin's disease.

Classification

a) Clinical

Since this disease presents different pictures which may run different courses, the need has been felt for an acceptable classification as a basis of comparison and as a guide to the understanding of the morbid signs and their development.

Numerous classifications have been proposed, some based on the most obvious clinical signs, others (more detailed) on the course of the various clinical or pathological abnormalities (Table 2).

Table 2. *Former classifications of disease stages*

REED (1902)	I = Lymph node enlargement II = Progressive cachexia	
LONGCOPE et al. (1920)	1 = localized form 2 = mediastinal form 3 = generalised form	} stages I and II
	4 = acute form 5 = concealed form	} stages II B and III
	6 = splenomegalic form 7 = osteoperiosteal form	} stage IV or special forms
CRAVER (1948)	Class I = localized disease Class II = regional disease Class III = generalised disease	

PETERS (1950)	Stage I = lymph node enlargement (single site)
	Stage II = lymph node enlargement (two or more adjacent sites)
	    A) without symptoms of generalised disease
	    B) with symptoms of generalised disease
	Stage III = involvement of two or more distant lymphatic sites and extranodal structures	

JELIFFE and THOMPSON (1955)	Stage 1 = lymph node involvement in only one main group
	Stage 2 = lymph node involvement in two or more adjacent groups, in either the upper or lower half of the body
	Stage 3 = a) generalised lymph node involvement
	    b) constitutional manifestations for which no other reasonable cause can be found
	    c) disease limited to retroperitoneal lymph nodes
	    d) involvement of structures other than lymphatics	

These classifications are primarily concerned with either the clinical course or the localisation of the disease. The classification of PETERS and MIDDLEMISS (1958) successively modified by KAPLAN (1962) is more in keeping with the several complicated forms now recognised and has been generally adopted (Table 3).

Table 3. *Present classification of disease stages*

PETERS and MIDDLEMISS (1958)		KAPLAN (Stanford, 1962)	
Stage	Involvement	Stage	Involvement
		0	no detectable disease (surgical excision)
I	single node or region a) local form b) stational form	I	localisation in a single node and adjacent structures
II	two or more groups of nodes, above or below the diaphragm, in adjacent sites A) without general symptoms B) with general symptoms	II	involvement of more than one region but in above or below diaphragm half of the body A) without general symptoms B) with general symptoms
III	two or more node sites, above and below the diaphragm A) without general symptoms B) with general symptoms	III	disease extends below and above the diaphragm A) without general symptoms B) with general symptoms
		IV	disease now generalized and demonstrable in: bone marrow; bone; lungs; more than one skin or subcutaneous area; gastro-intestinal tract as secondary; kidneys

Systemic symptoms or symptoms of generalized disease are: 1) otherwise unexplained fever, 2) night sweats, 3) generalized pruritus, 4) weight loss greater than 10% of normal body weight.

Other clinical signs are recognised but are not decisive of stage: a) malaise, b) weakness, c) fatigue, d) leukocytosis, e) leukopenia, f) lymphopenia, g) high ESR, h) skin anergy, i) alcohol pain. It should also be noted that liver involvement immediately indicates Stage III.

Recent practice makes lymphangiography an essential feature of clinical staging. This is used to visualise the involvement of the deep inguinal and retroperitoneal nodes during the course of the disease.

According to LEE (1966) this examination is not necessary in Stages I and II A, but is essential in Stage II B and thereafter, where 90% of cases present retroperitoneal involvement. This method always reveals a greater number of Stage III cases (from 35% to 50% of all cases, KAPLAN).

Table 4. *Lymphangiography*

Clinical stages	Distribution %	
	before lymphangiography	after lymphangiography
I	16	10
II	40	19.5
III	44	70

Lymphangiography contributes to the localisation of the involvement of deep nodes, but helps in a more precise stage classification too, somewhat changing the distribution of various cases (SCHWARZ, 1964—Table 4).

b) Histological

A completely different type of classification is based on the morphological features of the diseased tissue. The earliest, and formerly the most widely accepted of these classifications is that of JACKSON and PARKER (1947) (Table 5).

Table 5. *Histological classification* (JACKSON and PARKER, 1947)

1) Paragranuloma
2) Granuloma
3) Hodgkin's sarcoma

It is still of importance since it corresponds closely to the most commonly observed forms.

LUKES et al. (1963) re-examined this classification in the light of a large clinical series (377 military patients) with a view to introducing several factors leading to a closer association of the clinical, anatomical and pathological data: 1. localisation of the disease, 2. lymphocyte picture, 3. extent and distribution of sclerosis, 4. quantitative evaluation of atypical tumor cells. These authors, distinguish the following classes:

1. Lymphocytic and/or Histiocytic (L & H)
  a) diffuse
  b) nodular

2. Nodular sclerosis
3. Mixed
4. Diffuse fibrosis
5. Reticular

Table 6. *Histological classification*

JACKSON and PARKER (1947)		LUKES (1963)
Paragranuloma	I	Diffused lymphocytic and/or histiocytic form (L & H) (lymphocyte predominant)
	II	Nodular lymphocytic and/or histiocytic form (L & H) (histiocyte predominant)
Granuloma	III	Mixed form
	IV	Nodular sclerosis (formation of collagen)
	V	Diffused fibrosis (disorganised reticulum)
Hodgkin's sarcoma	VI	Reticular form

There are some points in which Lukes' classification approximates to that of JACKSON and PARKER (Table 6). The former is based on the presence of lymphatic tissue (Fig. 1) and conditioned by the shape acquired (Fig. 2) and by the quantity of histiocytes, Sternberg cells and connective tissue. The "mixed" type corresponds very well to the "granulomatous" form of JACKSON and PARKER and is distinguished by the polymorphous tissue pattern (Figs. 3 and 4). The last classes are those in which connective tissue (Figs. 5, 6, 7) or histiocytes (Fig. 8) predominate, the latter with tumoral features.

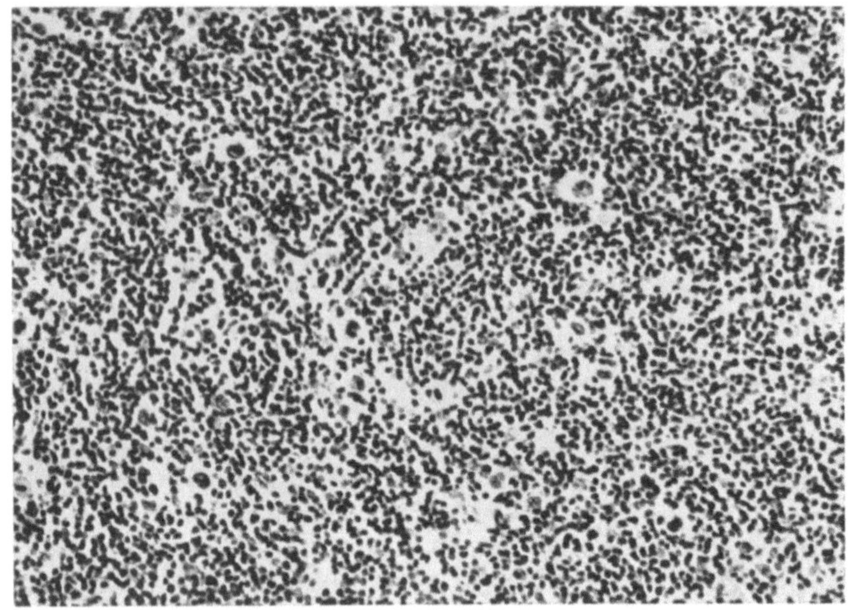

Fig. 1. C. T. no. 40 573—Hodgkin's disease. L & H diffuse (magnif. 180) Ist. Oncologia-
Torino

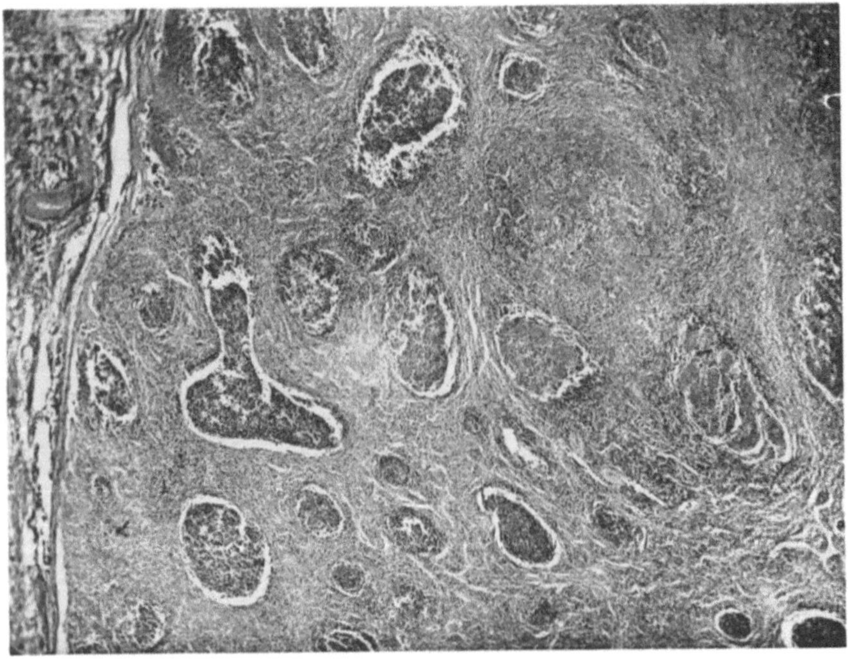

Fig. 2. C. T. no. 78 408—Hodgkin's disease. L & H nodular (magnif. 10) Ist. Oncologia-
Torino

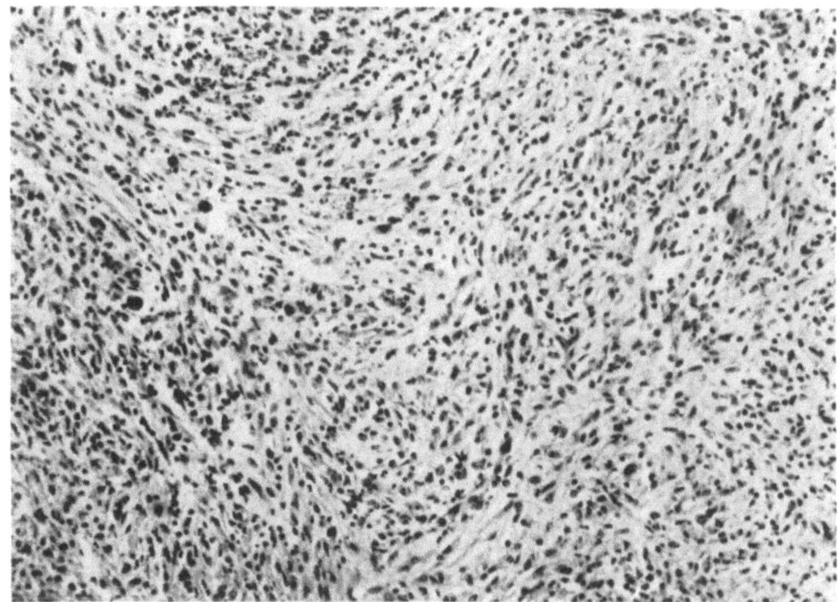

Fig. 3. C. T. no. 43 376—Hodgkin's disease. Mixed type (magnif. 140) Ist. Oncologia-Torino
Torino

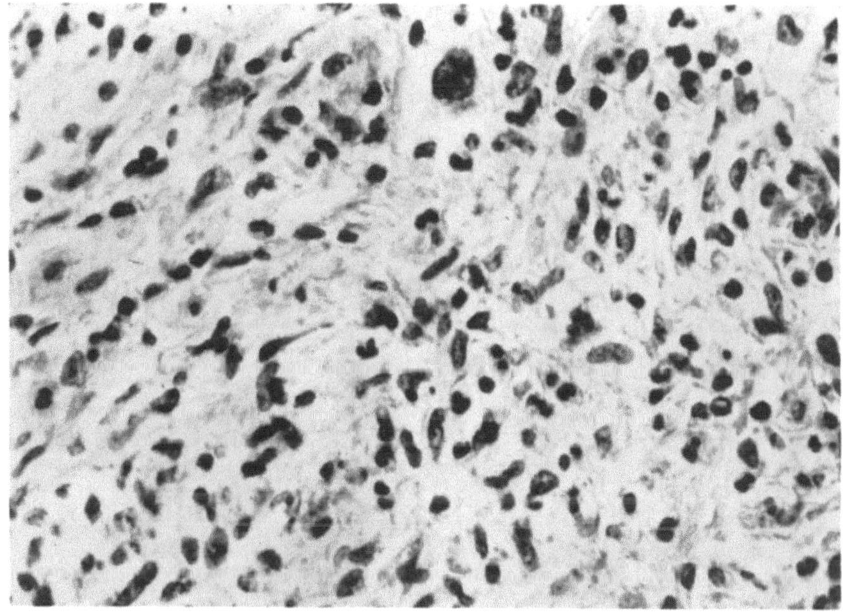

Fig. 4. C. T. no. 43 376—Hodgkin's disease. Mixed type (magnif. 530) Ist. Oncologia-
Torino

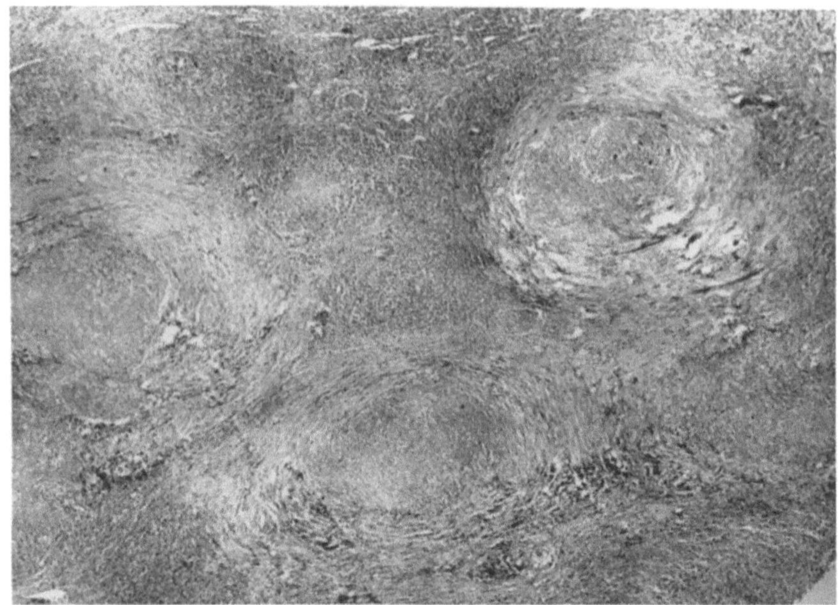

Fig. 5. C. T. no. 62 286—Hodgkin's disease. Nodular sclerosis (magnif. 20) Ist. Oncologia-
Torino

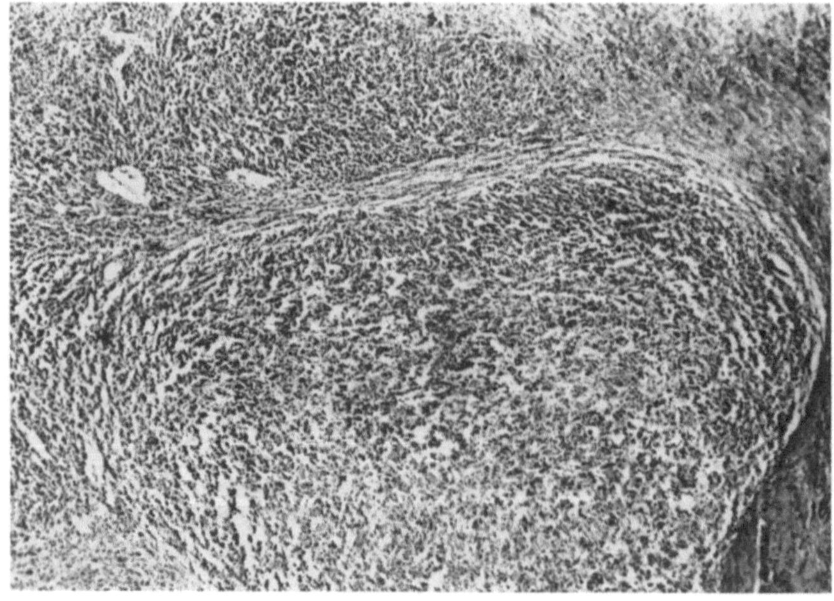

Fig. 6. C. T. no. 62 286—Hodgkin's disease. Nodular sclerosis (magnif. 70) Ist. Oncologia-
Torino

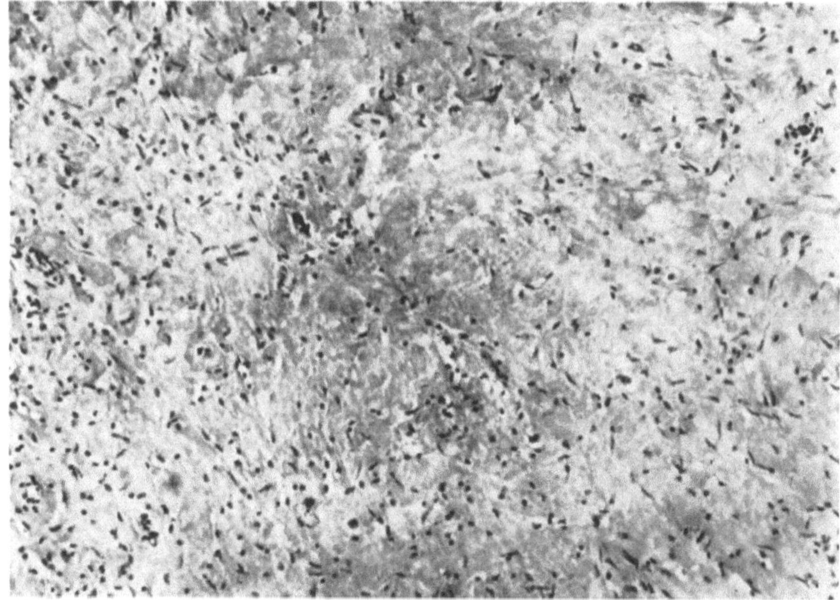

Fig. 7. C. T. no. 40 138—Hodgkin's disease. Diffused fibrosis (magnif. 140) Ist. Oncologia-Torino

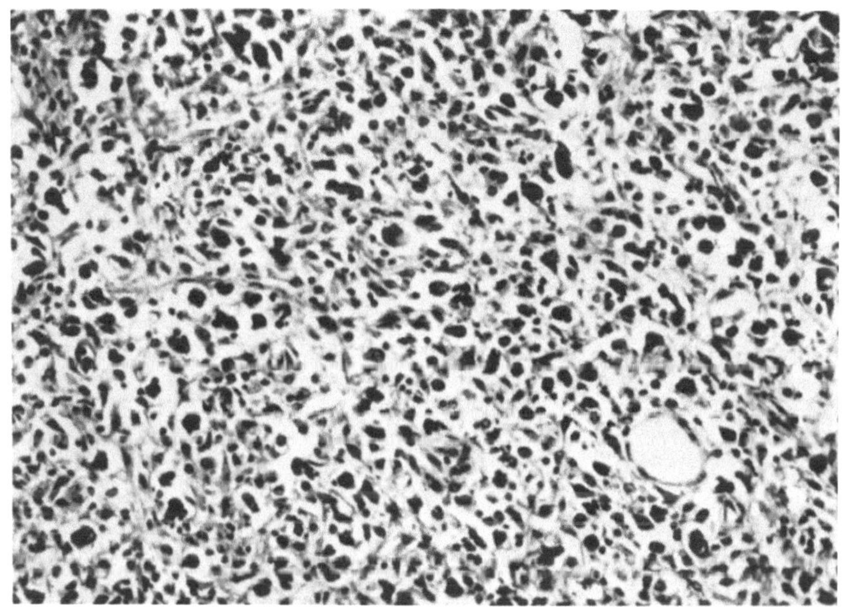

Fig. 8. C. T. no. 64 010—Hodgkin's disease. Hodgkin's sarcoma (magnif. 180) Ist. Oncologia-Torino (courtesy of STRAMIGNONI et al.)

In considering these data, it should be borne in mind that the series of LUKES et al. was largely composed of young subjects in whom the clinical course may not have perfectly corresponded with that observed in patients of other age groups.

The Natural Course of the Disease

Clinical course: typical features are: 1. painless swelling of nodes, unaccompanied by changes in the overlying skin, varying from the size of a small bean to that of a tangerine; 2. fever, often remittent, with apyretic periods, sometimes of Pel-Ebstein type; 3. pruritus, generally widespread, though sometimes confined to certain areas, occasionally intense and painful; 4. night sweating; 5. general malaise and tired-

Table 7. *Stage classification (according* KAPLAN) *with approximate 5 and 10 years survival (adapted from* KARNOFSKY)

Stage	Description	Example	Survival
Stage 0	no detectable disease (surgical eradication)	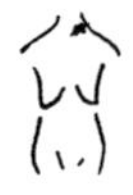	
Stage I	location to a single node or station and contiguous structures without systemic symptoms	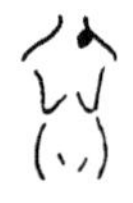	
Stage II	location to a more than single station or site, above or belov the diaphragm: a — without systemic symptoms b — with symptoms of generalized disease	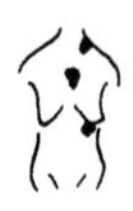	
Stage III	location on both sides of diaphragm plus liver a — without systemic symptoms b — with symptoms of systemic disease	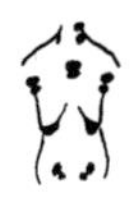	
Stage IV	location in several areas, besides lymphnodes and spleen: bone marrow-bone-lung-skin-pleura-liver-kidney-gastrointestinal tract as secondary	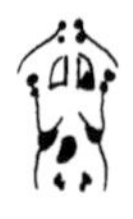	

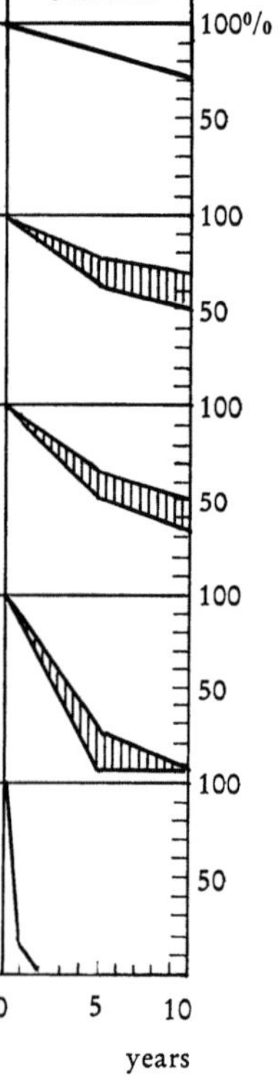

ness; 6. varying degrees of anaemia. These signs may not be concomitant and, in some subjects, the natural course may be difficult to recognise, particularly if the symptoms are successfully treated.

Onset may be insidious, with lymph node enlargement in one of the laterocervical or supraclavicular regions or, more rarely, in the inguinal region; careful observation will reveal slight, subfebrile temperature changes together with enlargement of the liver and spleen. In (nowadays rare) untreated cases, there is a progressive accumulation of symptoms, some of which eventually predominate. On the other hand, symptoms may be few and scarcely discernible over a long period.

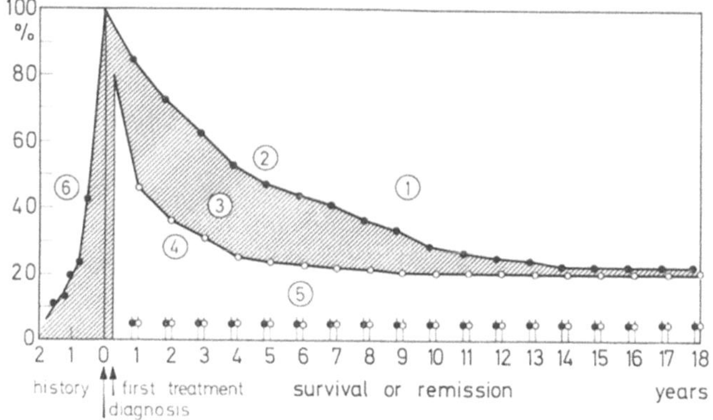

Fig. 9. Natural course of Hodgkin's disease primary treated cases (HEILMEYER and MUSSHOFF)

① deceased
② survival
③ living with recurrences after first treatment
④ remissions
⑤ remission after first treatment
⑥ % patients

Table 8. *Survival according to the histological classification* (STRAMIGNONI *et al., 1967*)

Histology	Authors	Year	Survival %	
			5 yrs	10 yrs
para-granuloma	SMETANA and COHEN	1956	77	—
	WRIGHT	1960	95	—
	HANSON	1964	94	44
	DI PIETRO and PIZZETTI	1966	35.7	16.6
	LUKES et al.	1966	73	44.4
	STRAMIGNONI et al.	1967	66.6	38.4
nodular sclerosis	HANSON	1964	87	56
	DI PIETRO and PIZZETTI	1966	47.1	9
	LUKES	1966	44.2	24.8
	STRAMIGNONI et al.	1967	36.3	7.4
granuloma	SMETANA and COHEN	1956	27	—
	WRIGHT	1960	27	—
	HANSON	1964	29	7
	DI PIETRO and PIZZETTI	1966	26.5	5.8
	LUKES et al.	1966	30.9	14.4
	STRAMIGNONI et al.	1967	18.6	5.5
sarcoma	SMETANA and COHEN	1956	0	0
	WRIGHT	1960	10	—
	HANSON	1964	0	0
	DI PIETRO and PIZZETTI	1966	13.5	0
	LUKES et al.	1966	23.8	4.7
	STRAMIGNONI et al.	1967	0	0

Some forms are classed as benign and present long periods of remission with comparative well-being, only occasionally interrupted by feverish episodes (DAWSON and HARRISON, 1961; C. I. E. WRIGHT, 1960). In the absence of external disturbing factors, these cases may run a chronic course in which acute episodes punctuate periods of symptomatological silence and well-being, though the latter become progressively shorter. Weight loss and malaise continue, fever becomes permanent and remittent-intermittent with occasional very high peaks. The pathological signs are often localised in one or more body segments and these clinical forms have been made the most important basis of stage classification. Progressive cachexia accompanied by anaemia and continuous fever forms the terminal picture. Survival varies from 1 year (in acute forms; some very acute forms are observed, ZOGRAPHOV 1961), through a mean of 3—4 years to 10—12 or more years in benign cases (Fig. 9, Table 8).

Special Forms

Several special forms are described (BOUSSER, 1966). Those with lymph node involvement as the only sign are rare, as are those with simple spleen or liver enlargement. Such forms are usually accompanied by fever and pruritus.

The so-called *mediastinal* form is characterised by increased deep thorax node size. Its particular and limited localisation in this site makes it clinically distinct; it usually runs a benign course and frequently presents a scleronodular histological picture (silent forms). Maximum severity of symptoms is uncommon; such symptoms include: dyspnoea, cyanosis, tirage, distension of neck veins, formation of collateral superficial circulation, thoracic dullness, pleural effusion. Many of these forms, however, are almost always attributable to invasion from a neighbouring site (i. e. the lungs) (RAMIOUL, 1960; STOLBERG et al., 1964).

Abdominal (splenohepatic or typhoidal) forms are typified by widespread abdominal pain, meteorism, constipation or diarrhoea as well as the fever, leucopenia and pruritus common to other forms. The appearance of lymphnodal masses with abdominal or retroperitoneal localization is generally considered a sign of unfavorable prognosis (CRAVER, 1964; WESTLING, 1965).

Primary *gastrointestinal* forms are relatively uncommon. Symptoms, only slightly apparent, include fever, gastric or intestinal pain, diarrhoea, sometimes vomiting, rarely intestinal obstruction due either to the primary localisation or to secondary swelling of lymph nodes.

The frequency of simple *pulmonary* forms has been variously reported as between 4% and over 40%. There are either mediastinopulmonary symptoms or disturbances of pulmonary and parenchymal function, sometimes at isolated sites (BOUSSER, 1966); these last are less frequent.

Localisation in any part of the *skeleton* is not uncommon in Hodgkin's disease (UEHLINGER, 1933; HARDER, 1960; PAPILLON et al., 1964) and will present as an isolated swelling, either with or without general symptoms, or as localised pain due to erosion of skeletal tissue.

Direct involvement of the skin *(cutaneous* forms), with progressive ulceration, is rare, though it may be the outcome of previous radiation therapy. Skin lesions attributable to scratching or ichthyosis are less rare; the latter may be aggravated by treatment.

Forms with *nerve* involvement are also described. Either the cranial or the peripheral nervous system is affected, though toxicosis of the central nervous system is occasionally encountered. Compression of the spinal cord due to invasion of the spinal space is more frequent.

Laboratory Findings

Anaemia is one of the most frequent features of Hodgkin's disease. Generally normochromic from the outset, it may become severe and haemolytic as the more advanced stages are reached; this is a common pattern in other tumor diseases. A positive Coombs test is encountered on are occasions, due to the presence of auto-antibodies; hypoferraemia, abnormal iron metabolism and poor utilisation of transfer iron are also observed.

Leucocytosis is present in over 50⁰/o of cases. Values commonly change slightly in response to treatment (ULTMANN et al., 1966, DEVOIS and DECKER, 1954).

Lymphocyte values are commonly depressed, particularly in the terminal stages or as a result of chemical treatment. Structural changes occur in response to PHA stimulation. Lymphopenia and lymphocyte depletion in tissue do not seem to be closely interrelated.

Increased *platelet*, levels classed as a typical sign of Hodgkin's disease.

Blood *eosinophile* increases have been reported since the time of the first clinical studies, though their significance is not fully clear. They are not always indicative of an allergen reaction nor a reflection of tissue eosinophile values (WAGNER, 1948).

There are few signs of increased *bone marrow* activity and aspiration rarely provides diagnostically helpful cells, though Sternberg cells are sometimes seen.

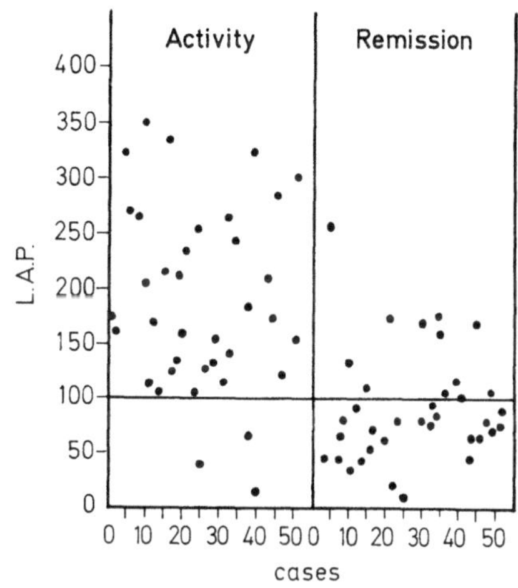

Fig. 10. Mean values of leukocytes alkaline phosphatase (FLURY and WEGMANN)

Leucocyte alkaline phosphatase values closely follow the course of the disease. High levels are observed in the active stage and low or normal values in both spontaneous and treatment-induced remission (FLURY and WEGMANN, 1964) (Fig. 10).

ESR changes are important in both diagnosis and prognosis. Rates increase when the disease is active and fall during periods of remission.

Blood proteins changes typical of this disease are also observed: decreased albumin values, attributable more to depressed production than to direct loss and primarily involving globulins, with increased α_1 and α_2 values (GOULIAN and FAHEY, 1961; MOESCHLIN, 1960), as well as increase in their glycoproteins, as in all inflammatory conditions. Increases in α_1 and *orosomucoid*, however, mirror the course of the disease since values fall to normal during remission or treatment (ANGLESIO et al.) (Fig. 11). Less importance is attached to high *complement* values (ROTTINO and LEVY,

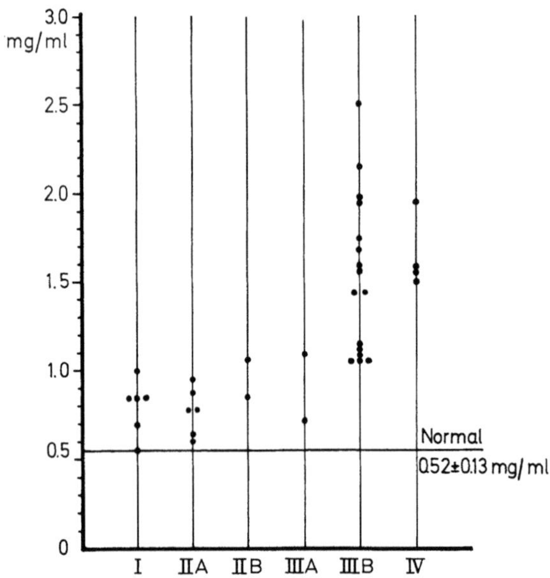

Fig. 11. Increase of orosomucoid values with progression of stages (E. ANGLESIO, A. CARBONARA, and G. MANCINI)

1959), to transferrin decreases and to the less imposing globulin (usually gamma-globulin) changes. In a small percentage of cases, *antibodies* increases are observed, but decreases are much more common, especially in the terminal stages. True hypo-gammaglobulinaemia, similar to that encountered in chronic lymphatic leukaemia, is rare (HOFFBRAND, 1964) and is then a feature of the advanced stages. Increased γ^M are equally exceptional. Increased *blood copper* is observed during the active phases (PAGLIARDI and GIANGRANDI, 1960) and is associated with increased serum haptoglobin and caeruloplasmin values.

Immunological status in Hodgkin's disease is singularly unlike that encountered in other diseases. Antibody and lymphocyte changes (commonly considered to be the components of immune reactions) do not reflect the observed clinical behaviour (ARENDS et al., 1964).

Of the circulating antibodies, gammaglobulin are in most cases normal and values are only slightly diminished (AISENBERG, 1966; GOLDMAN and HOBBS, 1967) except in the terminal stages. Hypergammaglobulinaemia and agammaglobulinaemia are rare (CROIZAT et al., 1961). Structural changes in these immunoglobulins have not been reported.

T. B. anergy has long been recognised as a characteristic feature.

In recent years, other skin reactions have been studied in an attempt to screen off previous contacts with T. B. antigens during youth. Skin reactions to purified protein (P.P.D.), Candida albicans, Tricophyton gypseum and measles antigens, as well as dinitrochlorobenzene, used as an example of a substance with which human contact is normally rare, all demonstrate the existence of a cell-mediated response. The *depression of delayed hypersensitivity* seems to be an important and constant feature of Hodgkin's disease and its diagnostic value has been emphasised, though its exact interpretation is still obscure (SCHIER, 1954; CHASE, 1966; CALCIATI et al., 1961; AISENBERG, 1966).

Chapter II

Surgical Treatment

Until recently, radical surgery was virtually ignored as a means of obtaining increased survival or even cure of Hodgkin's disease. Surgery was regarded as an ineffectual form of treatment, except as a means of palliation, and was employed for the removal of inconvenient swellings rather than in the hope of curing the patient. Biopsy was felt to be the sole motive for surgery and cases where satisfactory results followed radical excision of lymph nodes in single-site forms were attributed to luck rather than judgement. Splenectomy was carried out in cases of enormous enlargement but its outcome was felt to be uncertain.

To-day, however, surgical management of malignant lymphomas can readily be found in the literature and Hodgkin's disease has felt the benefit of this change of attitude (Table 9).

Various reasons have hitherto inhibited the use of surgery:

1. the disease was considered as a form of benign lymphadenitis;

2. many physicians turned to chemotherapy or irradiation and ignored the histological findings;

3. many surgeons excised only part of the lymph node for biopsy and did not carry out radical excision.

STORTI (1937) was one of the first to experiment with surgery as a means of treatment and obtained 8 and 15 years survival times in 2 cases.

Modern opinion, based upon the long clinical experience of many workers, can be summed up as follows: 1. Hodgkin's disease is a widespread disease of the reticuloendothelial system but involves only a single group of lymph nodes at the outset; 2. every effort must be made to ascertain whether the disease is limited to a single site; 3. the results given by surgery are permanent, whereas those derived from irradiation are progressive as tissues are in continuous changes. Up to 5 years, the two methods give equal survival rates; up to 10 years, surgery shows a definite advantage.

The operation must not be limited to the removal of a single node, as is done in many surgical departments. Radical elimination of the whole chain in the affected region (generally the cervical or supraclavicular region) must be carried out. Involvement of only one site is confirmed by: 1. chest X-ray, for involvement of mediastinal

Table 9. *Surgical treatment*

Authors	Year	Stage	Sex	Case no.	Treatment	Survival years			
						1	3	5	10
Storti	1937	I	—	2	surgery			1	1
Williams et al.	1951	I	—	1	surgery				1
Shimkin et al.	1955	I II III	—	7	surgery		4	3	
Marchal et al.	1956	I	—	4	surgery and radiotherapy		2	2	
Jackson	1956	—	—	3	gastric surgery			1	1
Rigat	1958	—	—	9	surgery				
Kolàr et al.	1958	—	—	14	gastro-intestinal			5	
Slaughter et al.	1958	I	—	10	surgery and radiotherapy			7	
Slaughter et al.	1958	I	—	8	surgery alone			6	
Becker	1959	I II	—	5	surgery	1	1	2	
Dawson and Harrison	1961	—	—	15	surgery				4(?)
End result group	1961	—	M	76	surgery			43%	
End result group	1961	—	M	61	surgery and radiotherapy			43%	
End result group	1961	—	F	61	surgery			59%	
End result group	1961	—	F	57	surgery and radiotherapy			34	
Smith	1961	—	—	3	surgery			3	
Rousselot et al.	1962	III	—	14	splenectomy			1	1
Lacher	1963	I II	—	11	surgery and radiotherapy			63.6%	
Kane	1963	—	—	1	gastric surgery				1
Monahan	1965	I	—	1	surgery				1
Molander and Pack	1966	I	—	74	surgery and radiotherapy		33.3	66.6	58.3%
Grace and Mittelman	1966	III	—	13	splenectomy	10	3		
Cornes	1967	I II	—	22	gastric surgery				
Cornes	1967	I II	—	21	intestinal surgery				
Schamaun	1967	I	—	1	oesophagus resection			1	
Schamaun	1967	I	—	1	lung resection			1	

nodes; 2. blood picture within normal limits; 3. spleen not palpable; 4. absence of fever and pruritus; 5. absence of lymph node involvement at bilateral lymphangiography. Unless these examinations are carried out and supported by clinical data, it is impossible to evaluate the indications for surgery (GELLER and LACHER, 1966).

Reference to surgical operation as a form of cure is to be understood as a procedure designed to prevent the spread of the disease by removing its initial site. If localisation is confined to the spleen, splenectomy can be performed under this head, as are cases of "hypersplenism" or residual enlarged spleen, which are doubtfully included.

Apart from the cases reported by STORTI, SLAUGHTER et al. (1958) have described a very instructive series of 18 cases (17 single-site, 1 with cervical and axillary involvement: in this last case, metastasis increased postoperatively). 13 cases survived for over 5 years' receiving only postoperative radiation treatment. In the 12 cases with laterocervical involvement, symptom-free survival periods ranged from 6 to 13 years.

The series of LACHER (1963) is not so conclusive. He compared survival rates in 11 surgically treated and in a larger group of irradiated patients (all in Stage I) and found a slight percentage difference in favour of the second group (63.6% as opposed to 65.6%); however, only 1 patient was treated solely by surgery.

Other results include: GALL (1943), mean survival 5 years in 41% of cases; R. D. WILLIAMS (1951), survival $8^1/_2$ yr (1 case); MARCHAL et al. (1956), 3.5 yr; DAWSON and HARRISON (1961) 10/15 recurrences between 1 and 10 years; PACK and MOLANDER (1966), 66.6% survival to 5 yr, 58.3% survival to 10 yr in 12 cases of radical surgery (3 neck, 3 axilla, 5 groin, 1 partial resection of the lung). The 10-yr survival value compares well with the mean value of 12.9 obtained with radiation therapy of Stage I cases.

Surgery is also favoured by the fact that Stage I, to which almost all these cases belong, includes "nodular sclerosis", a form which represents 15% of all the other forms put together (STORTI et al., 1965). Here, mean survival is 11 yr and there is a certain relationship between sclerosis and quiescence.

Digestive. Gastro-intestinally localised forms are also accessible to surgery. Exclusive localisation in the digestive tract is rare and this, coupled with the almost total or total lack of general symptoms, raises difficulties in diagnosis that may not be solved until an operation is performed (KADOSHCHUK and KUCHERENKO, 1964; COHEN and CANTER 1959; SCHULLER, 1966). Various workers (A. JACKSON 1957; JACKSON et al., 1959; KANE, 1963; COHEN and CANTER, 1959; KOLÁR and KACL, 1958; MAGGIORELLI, FALEG and PAZZAGLI, 1959; MARCHAL, MALLET and DUHAMEL, 1956; McNEER and PACK, 1962) have reported that, in the stomach, the lesion has the appearance of gastric ulcer and, in the intestine, may show the signs of an inflammation (often appendicitis) or threaten invagination or perforation.

In these cases, surgery is the treatment of choice. Survival times vary considerably, though a range of 5—10 yr is found in most cases since there is only one site, the removal of which is considered as a cure of the disease. Radiation therapy has little effect on the subsequent course.

Spleen enlargement is a well-known feature of Hodgkin's disease (i. e. splenic forms, KRUMBHAAR, 1931) and splenectomy provides a third example of surgical management. The most recent survey (GRACE and MITTELMAN, 1966) gives two indications for surgery:

1. Cases presenting with fever, spleen enlargement and absence of other important signs, if not of considerable anaemia. Diagnosis is based on histological examination of the excised spleen. Cases with exclusive localisation in the spleen run a favourable course (SYKE et al.; LONGO and BELTRAMI, 1958; STORTI, 1965; PACK and MOLANDER, 1966; GRACE and MITTELMAN, 1966). The situation does not present complications since the spleen is the most seriously affected organ and other signs are virtually absent. Such cases are rare: the series reported by AHMANN et al. (1966) includes cases in which the spleen had been completely replaced by lymphogranulomatous tissue or by very thin nodes (porphyroid spleen). GRACE and MITTELMAN suggest the following examinations: blood picture; bone marrow aspiration; erythrocyte survival; Coombs test; liver function (liver involvement is a contraindication to surgery).

2. Secondary hypersplenism. This is fairly common and is accompanied by pancytopenia, primarily severe anaemia with thrombocytopenia. Surgery is not strongly indicated in these cases and should be confined to those in which steroid therapy is impossible.

It should also be noted that here operative mortality is high (7—8%) and that results are not striking; survival times are not greatly increased and there is little improvement in the haematological picture.

MARCHAL et al., as well as STORTI et al. (1965) are definitely against this operation, and GRACE and MITTELMAN do not enthuse over the results obtained, for survival times ranging from 2 to 17 months in 13 reported cases and for the limited postoperative haematological results. The results reported by PACK and MOLANDER are equally modest.

GRACE and MITTELMAN also give a precise account of the surgical technique, to avoid gross trauma of the air pathways so as to prevent haemorrhage.

Splenectomy is thus of limited advantage in Hodgkin's disease, as opposed to certain forms of lymphatic leukaemia or reticulosarcoma. Extremely careful assessment of spleen activity must precede an operation giving such limited benefits.

Radiotherapy

Before their present differentiation, lymph node swellings were long considered as malignant tumours and, as such, subjected to the only reliable method of management, i. e. ionizing radiation. Hodgkin's disease was included and, since the beginning of the radiological era, such treatment has proved fruitful, both in the reduction of tumour size and in the progressive improvement of various symptoms, such as fever, anaemia, pruritus, malaise etc.

Radiotherapy in Hodgkin's disease has been further developed and some writers speak of a cure in the more fortunate cases (EASSON).

In some Centres, radiotherapy is still the sole means of management employed throughout nearly the whole course of the disease.

The aim of radiotherapy is to destroy lymphatic tissue and to block reticular tissue hyperplasia (CONGDON, 1966). There is progressive sclerosis of the residual connective tissue, which corresponds to a cure of the morbid process in the sense that lymph nodes become palpably smaller and disappear. Sclerosis, as is known, may start spontaneously and is greatly helped by a course of radiotherapy.

Cell irradiation seems to have a blocking effect on the flow of energy (BACQ and ALEXANDER), with biochemical interference with nucleic acid synthesis and mitosis; the latter reactions may depend on the effect of radiation on cell components containing information for DNA synthesis and cell division. In the result, lymph node size is reduced and immune response is blocked.

The physical effect of ionizing radiations is that of deep destruction of lymphatic tissue and Hodgkin's disease cells, as in the case of other lymphomas (KARNOFSKY, 1966). The salient features of radiotherapy are dose, distribution and field size (KAPLAN, 1968).

Early treatment seems to be very important for the success of therapy in radiology too.

The effectiveness of treatment is closely dependent on the total dosage employed (Fig. 12) and its distribution in time. The optimum dose rate is that which will produce tumour destruction with the least disturbance to tissue repair and reconstruction structures.

In Hodgkin's disease 200—250 kV have been used ("conventional" treatment-kilovoltage), with fairly satisfactory results (Fig. 13). At deep tissue level, there is a sharp fall-off of radiation dose and the best results are obtained in superficial lesions

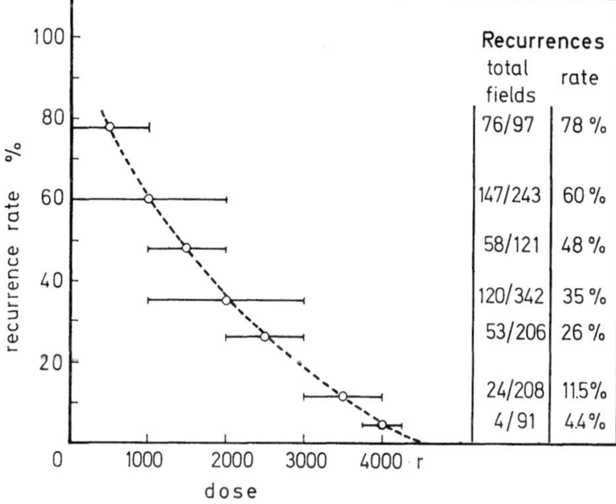

Fig. 12. Recurrence rates as a function of dose (KAPLAN)

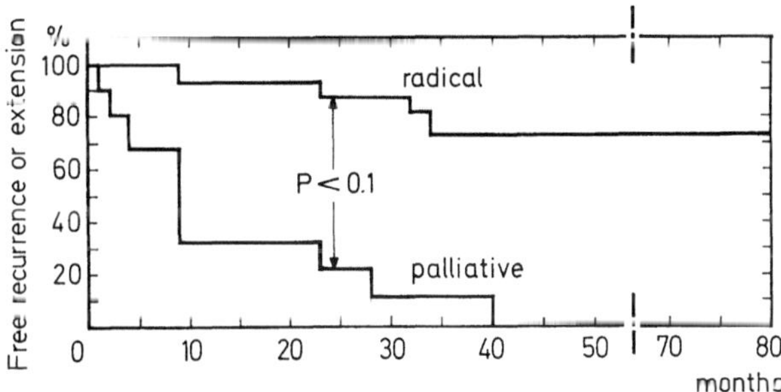

Fig. 13. Percentage of survival with radical and palliative treatment (kilovoltage). Hodgkin's disease. Stages I—II (KAPLAN)

(e. g. supraclavicular and cervical nodes). Fixed-field or cross-field irradiation is used, as required. Filtered hard rays are employed so as to spare the skin for subsequent treatments.

At first, total doses were limited to 800—1,000 r, according to tissue sensitivity, but today doses of 1,800—2,500 r per field, spread over 3—4 weeks, are employed (antiblastic treatment).

Good results are obtained, with the complete disappearance of lymph nodes (DEL VECCHIO et al., 1966) (Figs. 14, 15, 16). In the case of early or single-site forms, recurrences are rare and the disease appears to be cured; in any event, irradiation delays recurrences and gives some degree of remission.

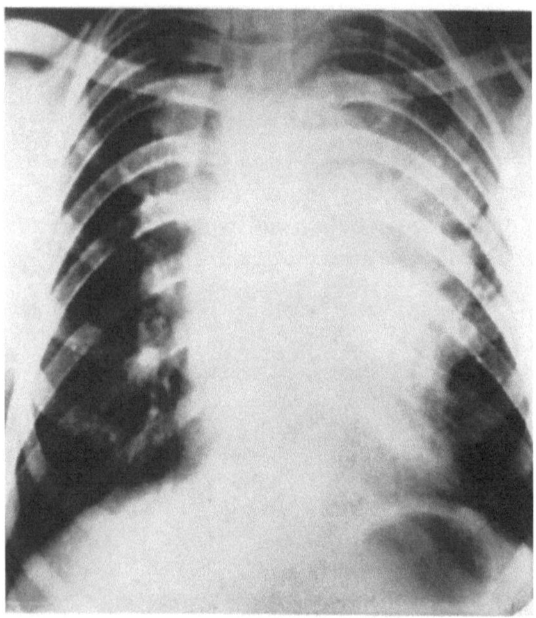

Fig. 14. Case G. G. Stage III, 9. 1. 1964. Mediastinal involvement-large shadow in left field.
Ist. Oncologia-Torino

High-energy (mV) radiation from cobalt 60, caesium 137 or linear or circular accelerators have been successfully used for deep lesions over the last 15 years (HARE, DAHLE and TRUMP, 1949). Depth transmission rate is much higher than with conventional methods; higher dose rates (3,000—4,000 r and over-megavoltage) can be delivered without damage to the skin and adjacent structures at the rate of about 1000 r per week. According to KAPLAN this seems to be a reasonably good estimate of the tumoricidal dose for Hodgkin's disease. Furthermore when more than an area is to be treated, the need to deliver doses as high as 4000 r to many areas involved makes it impossible to do it with conventional X-rays.

The field must be wide enough to include an adequate area around the lesion, since the disease does not originate in scattered areas but will, in most cases, predictably progress to adjacent areas (ROSENBERG and KAPLAN, 1966; HAN et al., 1967).

Although survival depends on many other factors, there is some relationship between the dose administered and survival times (KAPLAN, 1966; SCOTT and BRIZEL,

1964). The technical limitations and low doses typical of the beginning of the century readily explain the poor results achieved and the labelling of the disease as invariably fatal. If the tumour stage is accurately determined, a "cure" can to-day be claimed

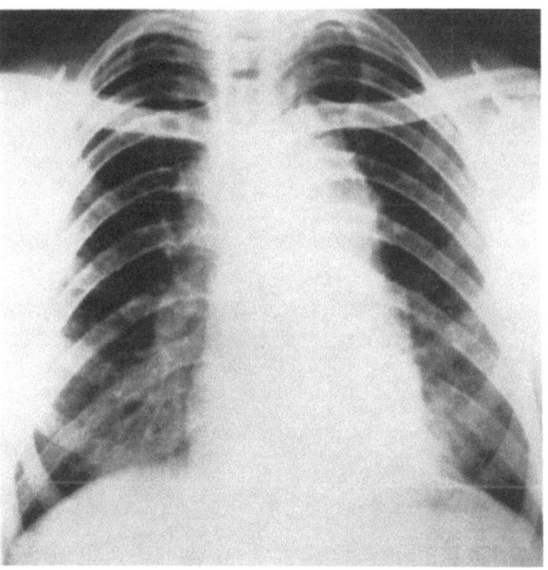

Fig. 15. Case G. G. Stage III, 12. 2. 1964. Reduction of mediastinal shadow during radiotherapy (kilovoltage) Ist. Oncologia-Torino

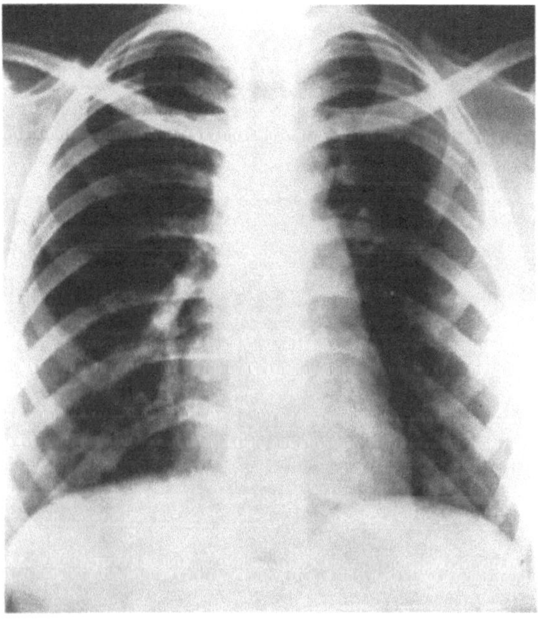

Fig. 16. Case G. G. Stage III, 9. 3. 1964. Cleared field after radiotherapy (kilovoltage). Ist. Oncologia-Torino

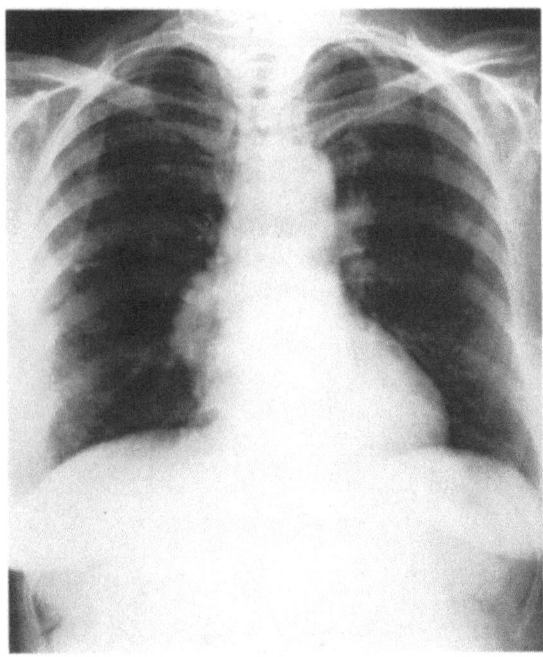

Fig. 17. Case C. M. Stage I, 30. 6. 1965. Mediastinal involvement right side. Ist. Oncologia-
Torino

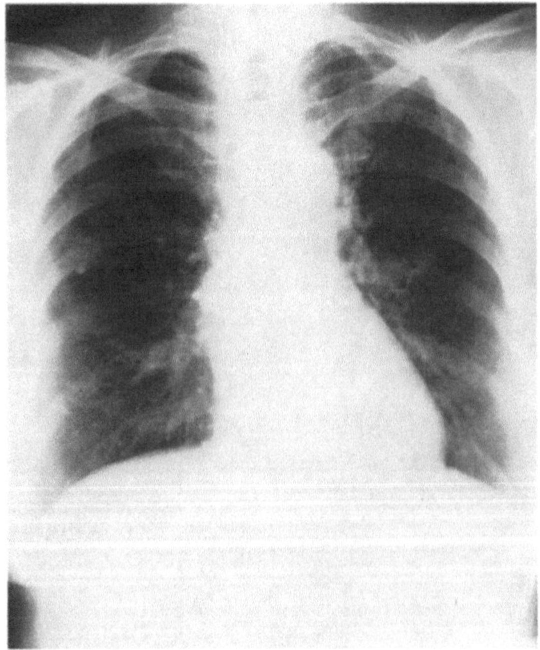

Fig. 18. Case C. M. Stage I, 21. 8. 1965. Mediastinal shadow reduced after radiotherapy
(cobalt). Ist. Oncologia-Torino

in a certain number of cases, especially early-stage local tumours (Figs. 17—18). In an idealised series of Stage I or II cases, with an average involvement of two areas, recovery may reach almost 90% of cases (KAPLAN, 1966), equivalent to an actuarial survival percentage of 82.4% (Fig. 19). EASSON maintains that it is possible to speak of a cure when, after a given post-treatment period (10 or more years), a group of patients is free from disease and has an expectation of life similar to that of normal subjects of the same age and sex. At present radiotherapy seems to be the only modality known to offer a significant chance for cure (KAPLAN, 1968).

The different techniques used are:

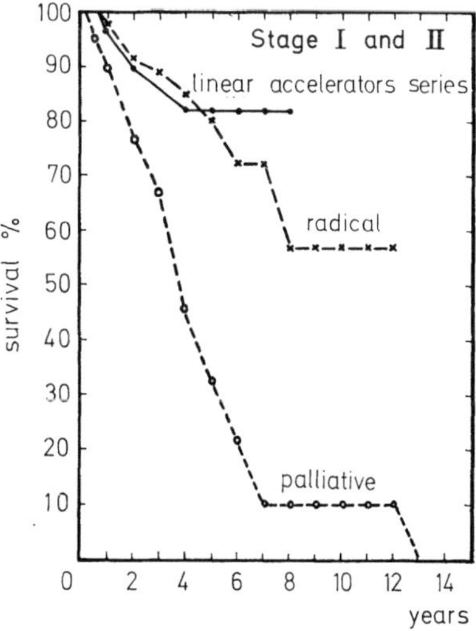

Fig. 19. Hodgkin's disease—localised forms. Actuarial analysis of survival in stage I and II; comparison of cases treated with megavoltage with those of kilovoltage, both radical and palliative (KAPLAN)

1. Local Radical Radiotherapy

The aim is to achieve ideal management of the treated field so as to eliminate the disease entirely (tumoricidal dose).

Doses of 2,000 r (conventional therapy) or 3,000—4,000 r (megavoltage) are used over about 4 weeks. The field must cover not only the main area affected (local field therapy) but also adjacent areas (extended-field therapy) in order to cover several groups of lymph nodes or a whole lymphatic chain.

This technique is the one now used in radiotherapy Centres and is suitable for single-site forms and to prevent the involvement of adjacent areas. Treatment should start from the most involved region and be completed before passing to the next. The plan of treatment must be adapted to the patient's condition, tumour localisation and stage. Relatively large subcutaneous foci and deep infiltrations of inner organs will clearly call for different approaches.

"Mantle-field technic" is special delivering technic to accomplish a large field irradiation in continuity to avoid missing some involved lymph nodes. It includes mediastinal lymph nodes, and during therapy care will be payed to protect lungs or glands (KAPLAN, 1968). Special maneuvres are recommended for mediastinal involvement.

Neurological complications may occur, compression to the spinal cord being the most serious. Irradiation of deep-lying organs is, in fact, open to discussion on account of the risk of complete or total cord section, with paralysis. Some authors (TUBIANA, 1966) favour low doses, others (GRIFONI et al., 1965) aggressive chemotherapy with high doses of NH_2 to prevent further damage of the spinal cord. The same remarks apply to mediastinal pressure and both situations indicate that management must be carefully chosen.

Marginal recurrences in adjacent lymph node areas are relatively frequent, whereas extensions are less common (JELIFFE, 17 marginal recurrences and 8 extensions in 25 cases). As already stated, adjacent areas should be brought within the ambit of treatment (Figs. 20—24).

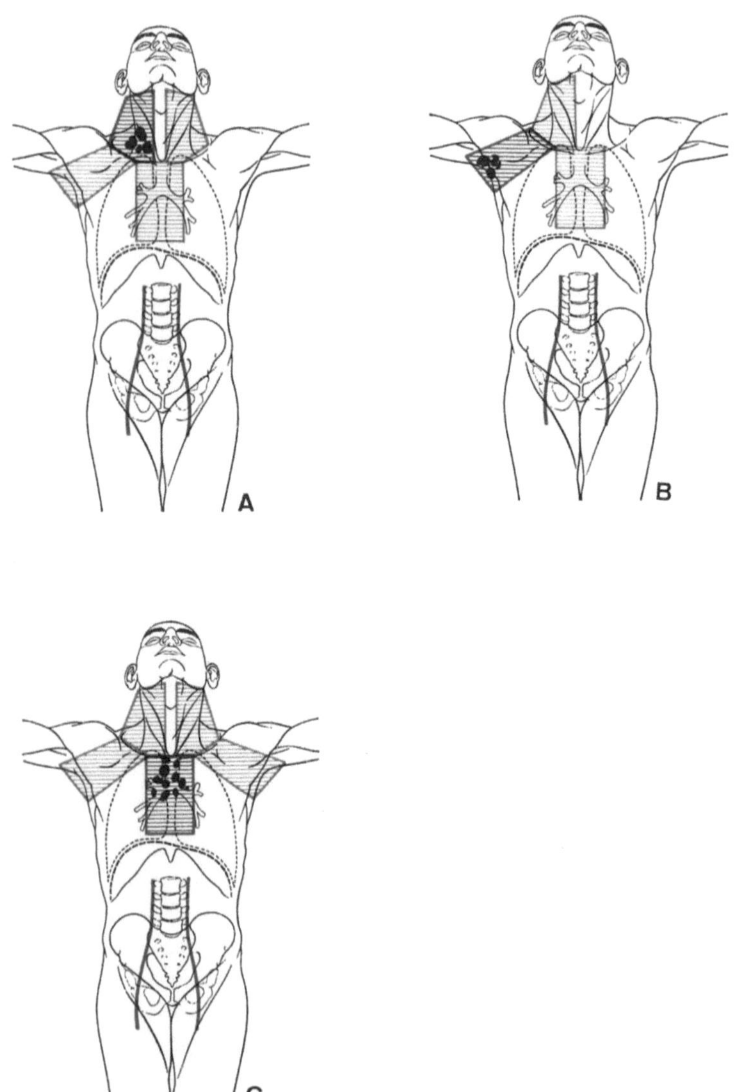

Fig. 20. Radiotherapy of Hodgkin's disease (FELCI). Stage I: involvement of lymph nodes in a single anatomical region above the diaphragm. A—supraclavicular, B—axillary, C—mediastinal; red areas, radical irradiation; blue areas, prophylactic irradiation

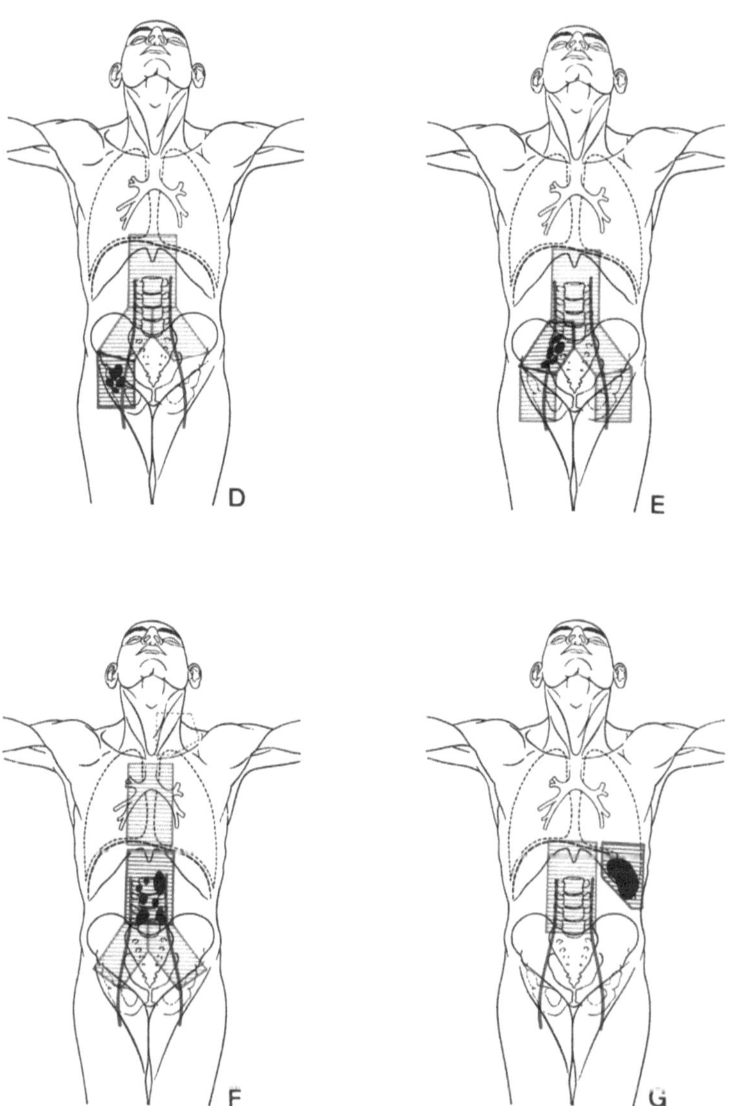

Fig. 21. Radiotherapy of Hodgkin's disease (FELCI). Stage I: involvement of lymph nodes in a single anatomical region below the diaphragm. D—inguinal, E—iliac, F—lumbar, G—splenic

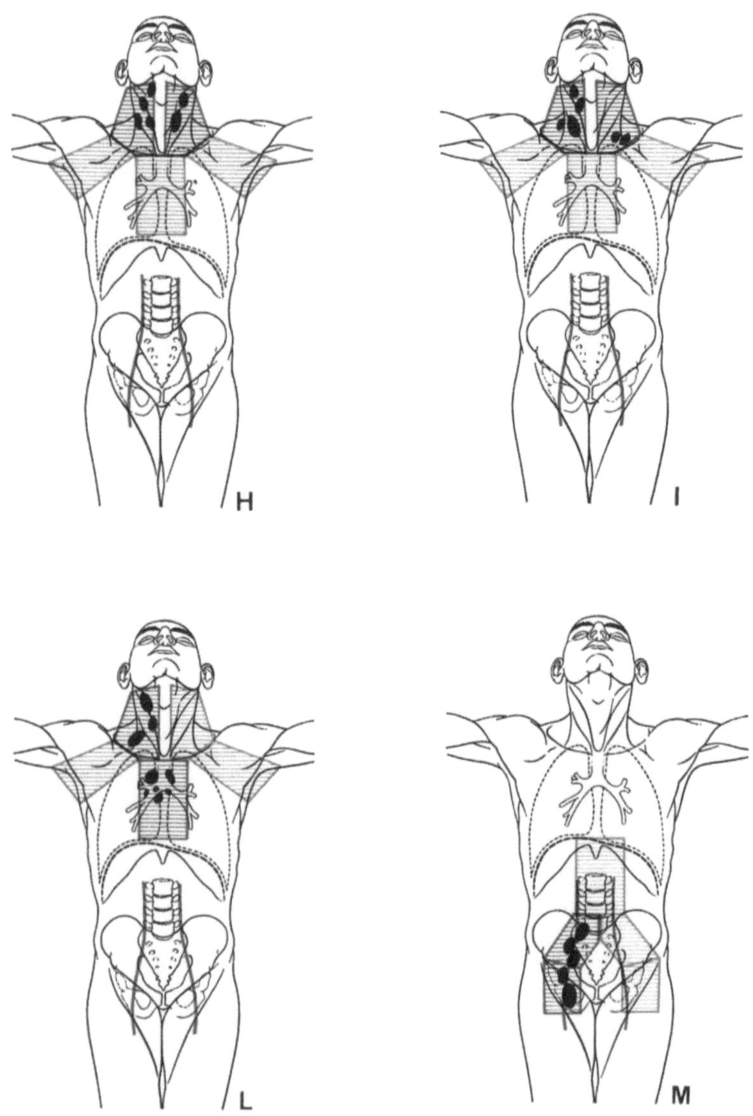

Fig. 22. Radiotherapy of Hodgkin's disease (FELCI). Stage II: involvement of lymph nodes in two proximal regions either above or below the diaphragm. H—cervical bilateral, I—supraclavicular left, both supraclavicular and cervical right, L—both cervical and supraclavicular right plus mediastinal, M—inguinal and iliac right

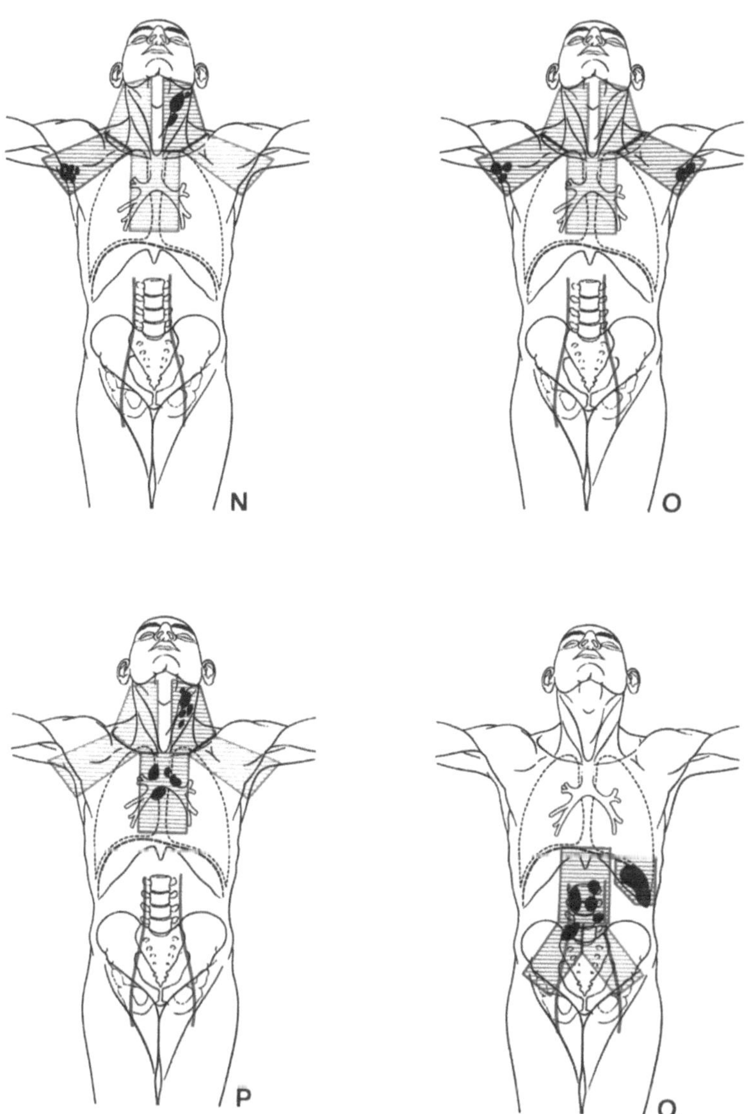

Fig. 23. Radiotherapy of Hodgkin's disease (FELOI). Stage II: involvement of lymph node
in more than two anatomical region or two non-contiguous regions either above or below
the diaphragm. N—cervical left, axillary right, O—axillary both sides, P—cervical left,
mediastinal, Q—lumbar, iliac and spleen

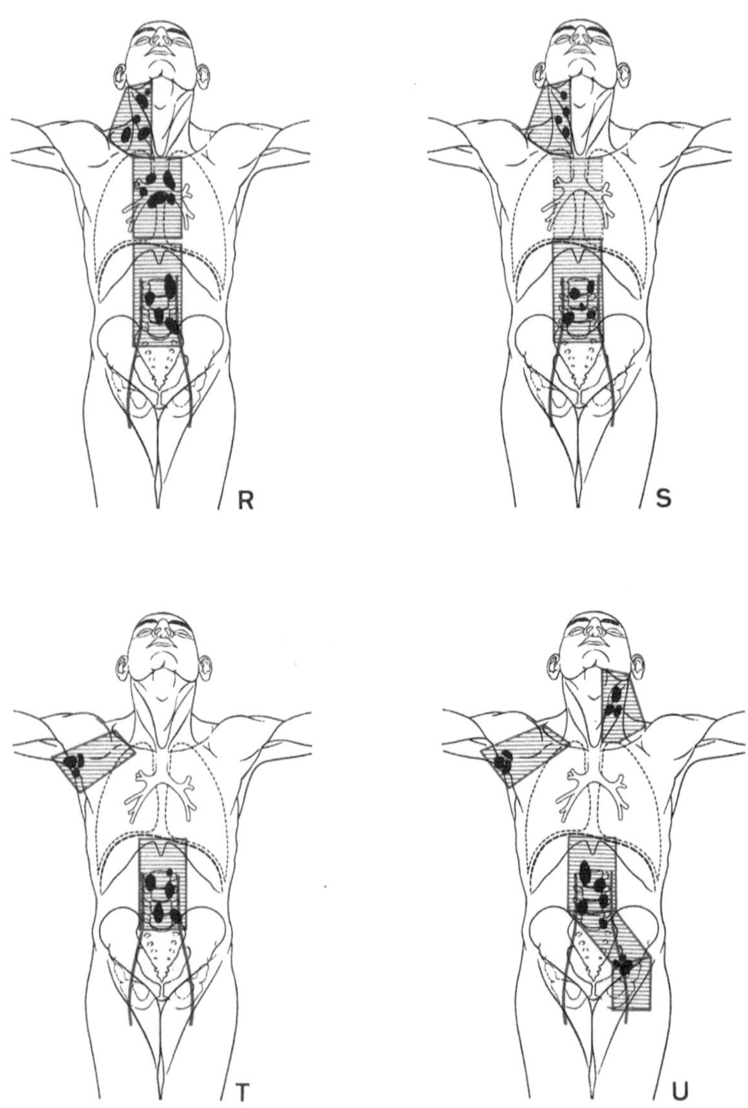

Fig. 24. Radiotherapy of Hodgkin's disease (FELCI). Stage III: involvement limited to the lymphatic organs (nodes, spleen, Waldeyer ring) of regions both above and below the diaphragm

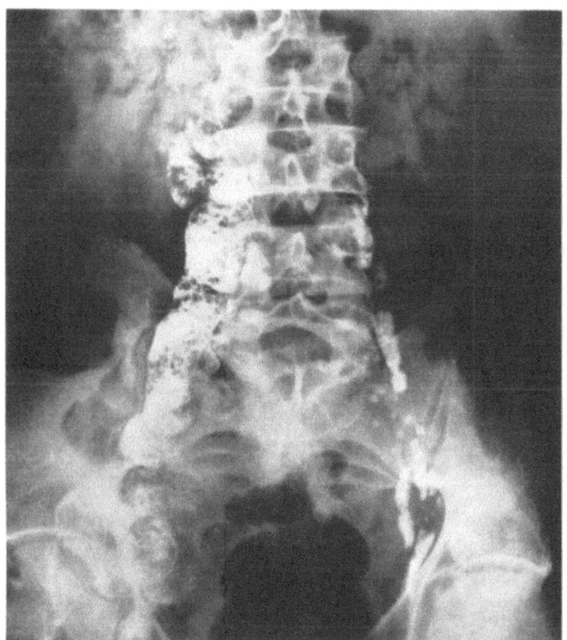

Fig. 25. Intralymphatic irradiation. Injection of Lipiodol F ^{131}I shows the enlargement of the left inguinal and retroperitoneal lymph nodes chain

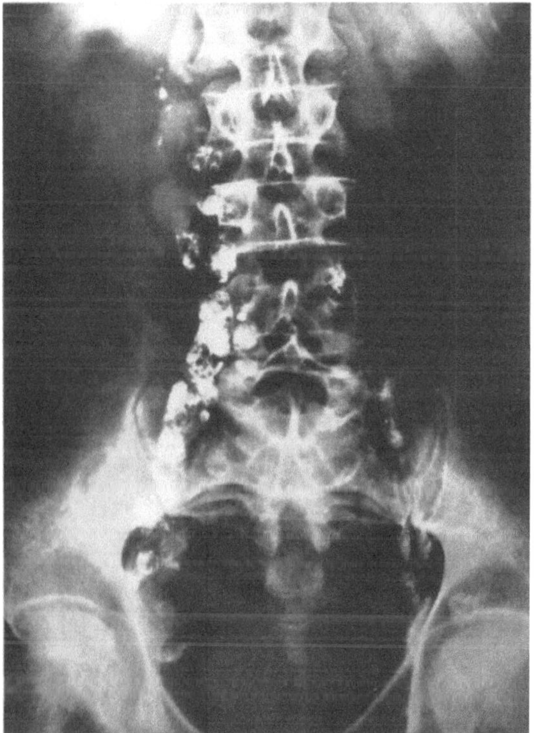

Fig. 26. Intralymphatic irradiation. Same patient since a 30 days period shows shrinkage of the lymph nodes (courtesy of CHIAPPA et al.)

2. Local Palliative Radiotherapy

This term is used to mean treatment intended to improve the patients' condition
in the advanced stages. It can be used in the case of Stage III and Stage IV lymph
node swellings on either side of the diaphragm, and spleen enlargement. Although
no remarkable success can be expected from this form of treatment, the results obtained by KAPLAN in Stage III and IV cases are worthy of attention. In these cases,
radiation was well tolerated.

Each Stage IV case (involvement of liver or other internal organs, skin or bone
marrow) must be considered individually. Treatment may occasionally include radiotherapy, though this will be limited to certain areas of the body; at the present time,
however, chemotherapy is the treatment of choice for many of these forms.

In pregnancy, radiotherapy naturally implies risk to the foetus but, unless a
(rare) inguinal form is involved, supradiaphragmatic irradiation can be carried out;
treatment of the lumbo-aortic chain must, of course, be avoided (VIRIEUX, 1966).

3. Total Body Irradiation

This technique was once favoured and was helpful in generalised phases of the
disease. To-day, however, chemotherapy is regarded as a better substitute (MELLI
and GRIFONI, 1960).

The total dose must not exceed 120—200 r fractioned over 10—15 days.

A similar form of treatment has been called "large-volume radiotherapy" (LEVITT,
1955) and involves a compromise halfway between local treatment and semiteleroent-
gentherapy; with respect to the former, its field is larger; with respect to the latter,
the irradiated volume is less. Unless an upper abdominal radiation bath is used,
paracentesis should precede treatment in forms accompanied by ascites. The method
is not free from disadvantages, however, and is generally considered old-fashioned.
Chemotherapy has taken its place and, though this is not without disadvantages of
other kinds, its benefits are undeniable.

4. Intralymphatic Radiation

CHIAPPA, RATTI and others have recently introduced a new irradiation technique
for the treatment of (mainly lumbar and inguinal) enlarged nodes. Iodinated oil
containing ^{131}I is injected into the lymph vessels and serves both for visualisation and
for therapy. Local activity from the beta-emitting source is well defined and clear
visualisation enables efficient external irradiation to be employed if the interstitial
treatment is inadequate (Figs. 25—26).

Chemotherapy

The most important weapon in the medical armoury against Hodgkin's disease
is chemotherapy, i. e. the use of substances having a cytostatic activity. These have
been in use since 1946 and are effective in the cure of tumours because they block
cell life. They are also known as antimitotics since they interrupt the mitosis cycle,
this being thought to be especially active in tumour cells.

From the theoretical viewpoint, these substances have signified the realisation of a dream, namely the sterilisation of the organism by means of medicaments. In practice, this form of treatment is helpful in those cases where irradiation is, as a result of metastasis or recurrence, no longer able to contain the disease.

Hodgkin's disease can be said to have been the proving ground for all chemotherapeutic drugs so far admitted into clinical practice. This has occurred because the disease is of a singular kind, its course is not especially acute and is readily controlled, and it has shown a favourable response to many of these drugs.

The substances employed differ in their chemical structure and biological action, as well as in the level at which their effect on the tumour is developed. They do not make an elective choice of neoplastic cells, but are active against any cell type in the reproductive stage. If uncontrolled, they can cause considerable damage to bone marrow, intestine and gonads.

Chemotherapeutic Substances

The main classification is into: a) alkylating agents; b) alkaloids; c) hydrazines; d) hormones. Each group has its supporters, reports of success, and special indications. Some have shown what is virtually a preference for STERNBERG tissue and have thus been the most widely used. Others have been abandoned after short periods of experimentation.

1. Alkylating Agents

This covers a large number of chemical compounds which are capable of combining with a number of chemical groups, many of which are important to cell life. In an aqueous solution, at physiological pH, they denature proteins, in particular nucleic acids. This is known as alkylation and kinetic studies reveal the replacement of a hydrogen atom with an alkyl group. Inactivation of biological systems follows this shifting or replacement of ions, and in vitro studies have shown that the DNA molecule is damaged to the extent that it is unusable by the cell, probably as a result of cross-linking, and that other cell components are also involved; such damage is similar to that caused by X-rays and these substances are called radiomimetics. To be effective against tumours, they must have two or more active groups in their molecule.

The following structural division of alkylating agents is recognised:

a) nitrogen mustard and its derivatives;

b) ethyleneimines;

c) sulphonic esters;

d) epoxides.

Not all of these are employed, though some are of fundamental importance, both clinically and experimentally, in Hodgkin's disease.

Two series are recognised: aliphatic and aromatic compounds:

1. *Aliphatic series.* This includes the basic compound, *nitrogen mustard*, this name being given to several substances. The classical example is (N-methyl-bis(2-chlorethyl)amine, also known as HN_2 (1).

$$\begin{array}{c} ClCH_2CH_2 \\ \qquad\qquad\quad {>}N{-}CH_3 \\ ClCH_2CH_2 \end{array} \qquad\qquad (1)$$

a) Nitrogen Mustard and its Derivatives

Nitrogen mustard is not only the first of these substances; it was for many years (and perhaps still is) the most efficacious. It is used in the form of a water-soluble chlorohydrate. Administration is solely by a venous or intracavitary route and a dose rate of 0.4 mg/kg is used. The solution deteriorates rapidly and cannot be stored. Contact with subcutaneous tissue must be avoided.

Administration is via venous drip, the substance being prediluted into a saline or glucose solution or (better) injected into the flow tube. Direct injection into a vein may cause thrombophlebitis following irritation of the walls. Doses may be aggressive (15—20 mg in a single injection), repeated on 2 or 3 days, or maintenance (3—5 mg on 5 or more consecutive days). Nausea and vomiting are common and presedation with anticholinergic or antihistaminic compounds or barbiturates is carried out to reduce these side-effects.

Toxicosis of bone marrow may be observed after 5—10 days. Depressed white cells and thrombocyte production is the main feature and will be prolonged and accentuated by the administration of high doses, though the condition of the patient, the stage of the disease and previous treatment are also important factors.

Other forms of damage include: irregular menstruation or amenorrhoea; alopecia (uncommon and mostly partial).

Bone marrow damage may be minimised in several ways; e. g. tourniquets, used to cut off the blood supplies to the limbs until 10 min after injection; marrow autografts; transfusions.

The therapeutic results of treatment are remarkable. Remission of fever, general toxic effects, pruritus and pain are followed by reduction of node, liver and spleen enlargement. Subjective improvement is also apparent (GOODMAN et al., 1946; JACOBSON et al., 1946; KARNOFSKY, 1965; DI PIETRO and GIACOMELLI, 1954; DAMESHEK et al., 1949).

If massive treatment is administered on account of the strategic localisation of the disease, morbid signs disappear and there is gradual remission of dyspnoea, compression and pain.

In general, the first administration or cycle is followed by regression of symptoms for a period of weeks, according to the duration of the disease, the clinical stage and the effects and intensity of previous therapy.

In Stage I or II cases (usually treated by irradiation), results are rapid and prolonged, especially in the absence of previous treatment. However, chemotherapy is more suitable for Stage III and IV cases, either as a primary or as a post-irradiation treatment.

There are, however, so-called "resistant" forms in which HN_2 produces a first remission (even where radiotherapy has failed) but the results are temporary or scanty. After the remission period, further irradiation may be carried out in some cases.

The particular side effects produced by HN_2 have been lessened in the case of other mustards, though these derivatives are slower-acting.

One example is *mannitol mustard*, 1,6-bis-(β-chlorethylamine)-1,6-desoxy-D-mannitol dichlorohydrate (2), in which mannitol (a carbohydrate) is bonded to active groups

$$
\begin{array}{c}
CH_2NHCH_2CH_2Cl \\
| \\
OH-C-H \\
| \\
OH-C-H \\
| \qquad {}_2HCl \\
H-C-OH \\
| \\
H-C-OH \\
| \\
CH_2NHCH_2CH_2Cl
\end{array}
\qquad (2)
$$

Mannitol mustard offers low toxicity and a therapeutic index of 50 (that of NH_2 is $= 10$). With this drug, leucopenia is less rapid, less intense and more readily normalised, interphase is lengthened, mitosis is blocked by chromosome damage and DNA synthesis is also blocked. As a result, cell metabolism is altered, with inactivation of enzymes and depressed cell activity.

Dosage consists of 50 mg (occasionally 100 mg) per day or on alternative days to a total of 800—1600 mg. Administration is by intravenous injection, though maintenance therapy includes oral doses of 50 mg once or twice a day.

Where the disease is widespread, results with mannitol mustard include frank reduction of node enlargement and remission of fever for periods of 6 mos. to 2 yrs. Hodgkin's disease is the most satisfactory field of application for this drug (SELLEI and ECKARDT, 1958; ESTEVEZ, 1964).

2. *Aromatic series*. These have been designed both to increase the aggressive potential of the mustards and to give fewer toxic side effects.

One of the earliest of these compounds was N,N-bis(-chlorethyl)2-naphthylamine (R 48). This is administered orally in doses of 50—400 mg per day (mean 100 to 200 mg). Gastric troubles are a common side effect.

It has been replaced by *chlorambucil* (3) (para[N,N-di-2-chlorethyl]aminophenyl-butyric acid), als known as CB 1348

$$
HO_2C(CH_2)_3 - \left\langle \underset{}{==} \right\rangle - N \overset{CH_2CH_2Cl}{\underset{CH_2CH_2Cl}{\big\langle}}
\qquad (3)
$$

Oral doses of 6 to 20 mg per day to a total of 400 mg are used. Tolerance is good and there is selective depression of lymph cells (chlorambucil has been employed with success in chronic lymphatic leukaemia). Results are slow and cumulative and, in the case of a first treatment, at least 1—2 weeks intervene before there is obvious improvement. Doses are initially high (15—20 mg per day) and are then decreased to maintenance levels (5—10 mg per day) for long periods (months). Side effects are rare though gastric disturbances occasionally lead to the suspension of treatment. Skin eruptions are even more rare. By comparison with HN_2, the effect on other white cells and granulocytes is slight, though leucopenia and severe thrombocytopenia may be encountered; such side effects are more frequent and more severe in previously treated (radiotherapy or chemotherapy) cases; they are often reversible.

Before the discovery of the Vinca alkaloids and other drugs, chlorambucil was considered good maintenance therapy in many forms of Hodgkin's disease, especially during relatively dormant intervals or on the occasion of slight fever or lymph node enlargement (GALTON et al., 1955; ULTMANN et al., 1956; BERNARD et al., 1957; DE VRIES, 1958; ROTTINO, 1957; MELLI and GRIFONI, 1960; ANGLESIO, 1958; ISRAELS et al., 1958).

Much use (not only in Hodgkin's disease) has been made of the transport form of NH_2, i.e. *cyclophosphamide* (B. 518) or N,N-bis(2-chlorethyl)-N,O-propylenesterphosphordiamine. This substance is thought to be liberated in active form by a phosphoramidase. Its formula (4) is complicated and enables molecule splitting to take place at the phosphoric bond.

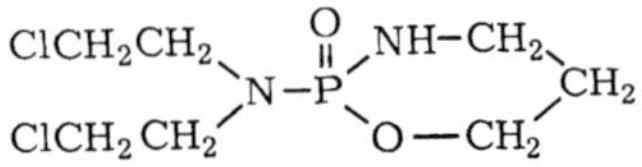

$$\text{ClCH}_2\text{CH}_2 \diagdown \atop \text{ClCH}_2\text{CH}_2 \diagup \text{N} - \overset{\overset{\text{O}}{\|}}{\text{P}} \underset{\diagdown \text{O} - \text{CH}_2}{\overset{\diagup \text{NH} - \text{CH}_2 \diagdown}{}} \text{CH}_2 \diagup \qquad (4)$$

Intravenous (sometimes intramuscular) injections of 100—200 mg per day are given. Maintenance therapy makes use of 50 mg tablets (2—3 per day). Totals of 5—7 g. may be reached and tolerance is good over long periods. Leucopenia and anaemia are important sequelae, both the myeloid and the lymphatic white cells being involved.

Side effects are not uncommon and include: alopecia, sometimes total and irreversible, haemorrhagic cystitis, gastric disturbances and (rarely) skin eruptions.

Good results have been obtained in many cases and long periods of remission have been reported (GERHARTZ, 1964; GROSS and LAMBERS, 1958; KOPP and HEINECKER, 1965; LASZLO, 1962; FAIRLEY et al., 1966).

The incorporation of some biological-like substances, such as aminoacids, has improved the effectiveness of some compounds, such as the phenylalanine derivatives. These have been used in several diseases, including Hodgkin's disease, mostly in East Europe. The prototype was para-di(2-chlorethyl)aminophenylalanine. The L form is the most active; the DL form *(sarcolysin)* is also used on occasions.

WILKINSON et al. (1963) reported success in lymphatic diseases, including Hodgkin's disease, with an association of an HN_2 derivative and uracil, urchlorethamine or *uromustine* (a 5-bis[chlorethyl]aminouracil). This compound is not much used. Administered orally, its effects are similar to those of HN_2, but tolerance is improved, local toxic damage is small and its action is both rapid and prolonged (LANE et al., 1960).

b) Ethyleneimines

Some members of this group were used with success at the beginning of the chemotherapy era. The first of the series was 2, 4, 6, triethylenimine-S-triazine, also called *triethylene-melamine* or TEM (5). Oral administration (2.5 mg) is almost always used. Problems of dosage and absorption have led to its falling into disfavour. It is preferably taken in the morning, after fasting, in association with sodium bicarbonate to ensure absorption in an inactive form followed by slow transformation to the active quaternary form. Dosage of 2.5 mg per day for 3 days is recommended

(RUNDLES, 1958) Patient sensitivity (low, medium or high) is based on leucocyte response and toxic effects on the digestive system. Maintenance doses of 0.5—1 mg at intervals of 2—5, 5—10 or 7—14 days are suggested.

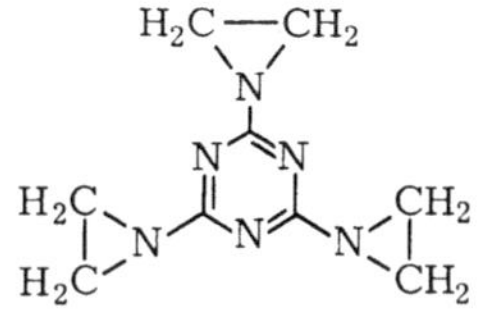

$$H_2C—CH_2 \quad \text{(triethylenemelamine structure)} \tag{5}$$

Side effects are less common than with nitrogen mustard, though marrow disturbances are more serious since cytopenias are readily provoked.

On the other hand, inhibition of node enlargement, fever and general symptoms is good and similar to that obtained with nitrogen mustard and its derivatives (KARNOFSKY et al., 1951; BJERRE HANSEN and BICHEL, 1951; PATERSON et al., 1953). For these reasons, and for its ease of administration, TEM has been used for prolonged treatment (ROTTINO et al., 1952; BOND et al., 1959; SILVERBERG et al., 1952).

Therapeutic results with TEM are soon apparent, whereas toxic effects are delayed on account of accumulation. Leucopenia or thrombocytopenia is therefore almost inevitable, because the onset is unpredictable. WRIGHT claims that levels will fall between the 5th and the 23rd treatment day, but individual tolerance varies considerably.

A second product of this series is triethylenethiophosphoramide (Thio TEPA). This is less toxic than TEM but less active. Its formula is similar to that of TEM (6).

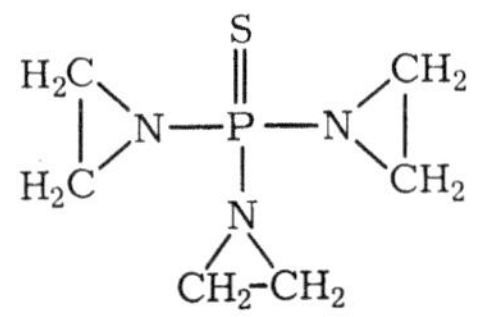

$$\text{(triethylenethiophosphoramide structure)} \tag{6}$$

Thio TEPA is administered intravenously in doses of 10—20 mg (total 300 to 400 mg). Individual tolerance varies greatly. The compound can be directly injected into the tumour, but intracavitary injection in the case of peritoneal or pleural effusion is more common. Side effects are few, though leucopenia is a principal sequela.

Clinical experience has shown that Thio TEPA, which is active against malignant tumours, is able to give useful results (sometimes complete regression) in Hodgkin's disease. Results are not longlasting, however, and prolonged treatment is advised. Success patterns vary greatly, however (ULTMANN et al., 1966).

Another derivative in this series is 2,3,5 trisethyleneiminobenzoquinone. This was derived from another compound, E 39 (2.5-bis(ethyleneimine)3 6 dipropioxy-1-4-

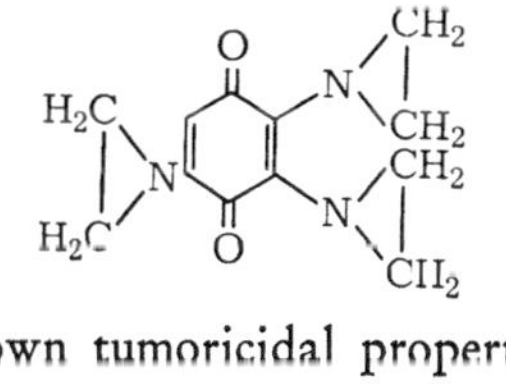

$$\text{(trisethyleneiminobenzoquinone structure)} \tag{7}$$

benzoquinone) which had shown tumoricidal properties in vitro and in vivo. *Trisethyleneiminobenzoquinone* (7) contains a benzole ring with cytostatic properties. To this, 3 ethyleneimine groups are bonded.

This substance is water-soluble. Dosage is 0.2 mg daily (to totals of 3—5 g), intravenously; oral doses are higher (0.5 mg) (total 4—6 g). In both cases, tolerance is good, though marrow damage is not inconsiderable. Handling is easy, though care must be taken to avoid thrombophlebitis.

LINKE used this substance on 134 patients, with 96 good, 21 slight and 17 nil results (the last being cases in advanced stages). In general, results are good since administration can be protracted with an attack dose (intravenous) and oral maintenance doses; in this way, radiotherapy may be employed contemporaneously or afterwards.

c) Sulphonic Acid Esters

A sulphonic ester, whose activity appears to be limited to certain non-lymphomatous disease (GALTON et al., 1958), *busulphan* (1,4-dimethane sulphonyloxybutane) has given poor results in the treatment of Hodgkin's disease.

d) Epoxides

These have alkylating properties but are very seldom used; *diepoxypiperazine* (N,N'-bis(2,3-epoxy-n[propyl]piperazine) has been administered intravenously with some success in Hodgkin's disease.

2. Alkaloids

There are many alkaloid substances, some of which have the property of arresting mitosis in the metaphase.

The oldest known of these substances is *colchicine*. This may be administered orally or intravenously and is used (infrequently) as an F substance (desacetyl-methylcolchicine) in tumour therapy (GROLLMAN et al., 1955). Its molecule has 3 benzoic rings (8).

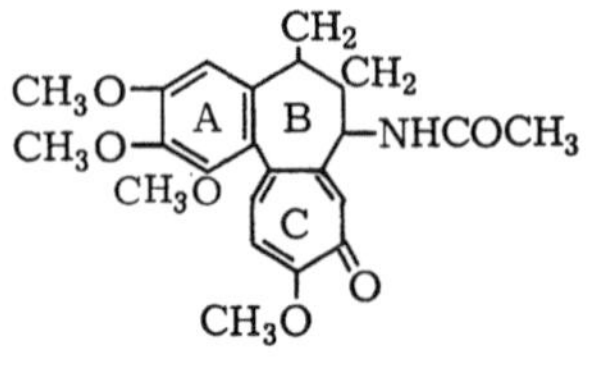

$$\text{CH}_3\text{O}\!\!-\!\!\overset{\displaystyle \text{CH}_2}{\underset{\text{CH}_3\text{O}}{\boxed{\text{A}}\ \boxed{\text{B}}}}\overset{\text{CH}_2}{-}\text{NHCOCH}_3 \qquad (8)$$

Doses of 2—5 mg per day to a total of 40—50 mg are employed; reduction of lymph node and spleen enlargement and of fever, together with general symptomatic improvement, are observed. Toxicity is high, however, and this led to experiments with the readily soluble d-tartrate salt of the methyl ester of trimethylcolchicinic acid. Good clinical results were obtained, but the margin of safety between the toxic and the therapeutic dose was too small and the substance has now been almost abandoned.

Greater success has been obtained with alkaloids of Vinca rosea (Catharanthus roseus). The most important at the moment are *vincaleucoblastine* (VLB) and *vincrystine* VCR) (9).

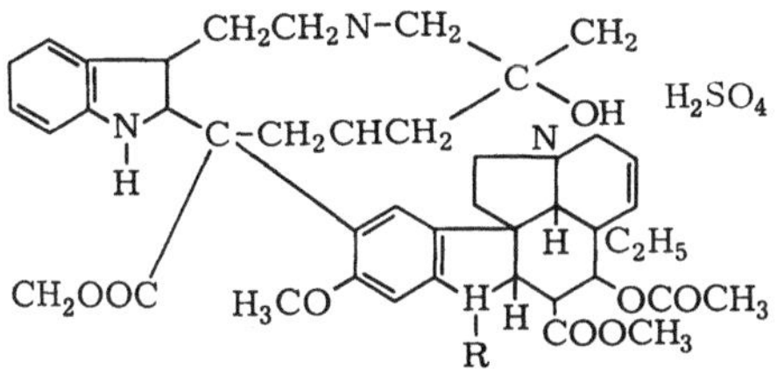

$$\text{VBL–R} = CH_3 \qquad \text{VCR–R} = CHO \qquad (9)$$

These substances are readily soluble in water and are administered intravenously at doses of 10—15 mg per week (VLB) or 1—2 mg per week (VCR). Solutions must be freshly prepared. Both substances have been successful in the treatment of malignant lymphoma; in Hodgkin's disease, VLB has given the best results. It has the typical spindle-inhibiting effect and arrests division in the metaphase, giving rise to C-mitosis (MARMONT et al., 1964). The formulae of VLB and VCR are similar, though the latter has a formyl group; the general pattern is that of a dimer alkaloid containing an indole and a dihydroindole group (SVOBODA, 1966). The mechanism of action is in both cases exercised by means of an interference with critical points in mitosis (BIESELE, 1958), the effects varying with high and with low doses (LETTRÉ, 1966). Spindle formation is affected by the creation of disulphur bridges in the long fibrous molecules. VLB may interfere with glutammic acid; this would explain its antimetabolic action. At low concentrations, spindle block is accompanied by duplication of chromosomes, but there is no separation into chromatids. At higher concentrations, chromosome lesion occurs, there is coalescence and shrinkage of the spindle, leading to the so-called "ball metaphase".

The treatment of haemoblastosis and many other diseases with VLB has helped to make it one of the treatment of choice for Hodgkin's disease. Here, positive response to treatment is high (15— 90% of cases), even in forms that have proved resistant to other types of therapy.

The effects of the drug are quickly apparent; in this, it is different from colchicine, which it otherwise resembles in many ways. The first sign is a general feeling of well-being, possibly due to reduction of toxicosis. Symptoms, and node enlargement, gradually regress. Body weight increases and more or less normal conditions are restored. These results can be maintained by continuous treatment over long periods and are similar to those obtained with other drugs (MATHÉ et al., 1962; MARSDEN, 1963; OBRECHT et al., 1964; GARY-BOBO, 1966; KEISER et al., 1962; ARMSTRONG et al., 1962).

Side effects are relatively few: depressed WBC after 10 days; granulocyte levels are most affected, followed by the slower proliferating lymphocytes. Red cells and thrombocytes are scarcely affected; here again the drug differs from colchicine. Leucocyte values usually return to normal within 8—15 days, though WBC and granulocyte values may occasionally remain low, especially if there has been damage to bone marrow from previous therapy. It is uncertain whether VLB is specific for pathological tissue, though this is gradually damaged and swellings disappear (MARMONT et al., 1964).

A transitory rise in temperature may be observed on the first post-injection day. This has no effect on the therapeutic result.

Nausea is very rarely seen; there are practically no reports of alopecia. On the other hand, depression, hallucinations and peripheral neuritis may be encountered (VAITKEVICIUS et al., 1962; KEISER, 1962). If the solution enters the subcutaneous tissue, local irritation may be caused and last for days or even weeks.

VLB can, therefore, be classed as a leading chemotherapeutic drug in the treatment of Hodgkin's disease. It is true that it has much the same advantages as the alkylating agents. In addition, it is better tolerated, marrow damage is slight (BICHEL, 1966) and the resulting leucopenia is easily reversible. In some forms, where there is marrow exhaustion, prolonged steroid treatment can be avoided (MARMONT and FUSCO, 1964).

Treatment with VCR alone, however, has not brought the same degree of success. Reported cases are very few and the results are only slight and of short duration (MATHÉ et al., 1962; SVOBODA, 1966). Association of the two alkaloids, by contrast, has been found useful in cases that have resisted previous treatment. Doses of 10 mg VLB and 0.4 mg VCR are used, though it is not known which of the two drugs is more active nor the tissue component affected. Clinical experimentation is still incomplete and the duration of results is as yet uncertain.

VCR is easily administered and well-tolerated. Doses of 1—2 mg per week are injected intravenously. The mechanism of action seems to be different from that of VLB, though it is known to block mitosis in the metaphase. Its behaviour with respect to haemopoietic tissue is also different and this fact, together with the greater frequency of neurological complications, including pain and paralysis, suggests that it has a different point of attack. Among its side effects, reversible alopecia should be noted.

3. Hydrazine Derivatives

The latest chemotherapeutic product, *methylhydrazine,* is the result of the studies of BOLLAG et al. on the inhibition of experimental tumours. The first clinical studies (D'ALESSANDRI, 1963; MARTZ et al., 1963) showed it to be of particular help in the treatment of Hodgkin's disease and their results have since been many times confirmed (MATHÉ et al., 1964; KUMMER et al., 1965; TODD, 1965; BRUNNER and YOUNG, 1965; KENIS et al., 1965; FAZIO et al., 1965; OBRECHT at al., 1966; BACKHOUSE et al., 1966; SICHER et al., 1965; SARTORIS et al., 1968; ANGLESIO, 1965; WITTE et al., 1966; BERNARD, 1966; FAIRLEY et al., 1966; HANSEN et al., 1966).

Methylhydrazine is the chlorhydrate of 1-methyl-2p(isopropylcarbamyl)benzyl-hydrazine and is available in tablets (50 mg) or vials (250 mg) for intravenous use. The formula is (10):

$$\text{CH}_3\text{HNHCH}_2 - \langle \bigcirc \rangle - \text{CONH} - \text{CH} \big\langle \begin{smallmatrix} \text{CH}_3 \\ \\ \text{CH}_3 \end{smallmatrix} \ -\text{HCl} \tag{10}$$

The action of the drug is not known, though it is assumed to be different from the other chemotherapeutics already mentioned. It depresses mitosis by prolonging the interphase. The formation of oxidation products and the liberation of peroxides and hydroxides which, in vitro, degrade DNA and cause the formation of chromosome bridges (BERNEIS et al., 1965; ZELLER et al., 1963; WEITZEL et al., 1964), make its action similar to that of ionizing radiations.

Success with methylhydrazine in the treatment of Hodgkin's disease has been confirmed on many occasions and percentages as high as 60% have been reported. Being a newcomer, however, its successes may be due to the fact that the cases treated were those in which survival rates are high. On the other hand, some workers report rapid results in cases where the drug was the first therapy used and in others which had resisted previous treatment (Figs. 27—29). It does not display cross-resistance with other products and can be used either alone or in association with other forms of therapy (D'ALESSANDRI et al., 1963; HAMMER, 1967; WAGNER et al., 1965).

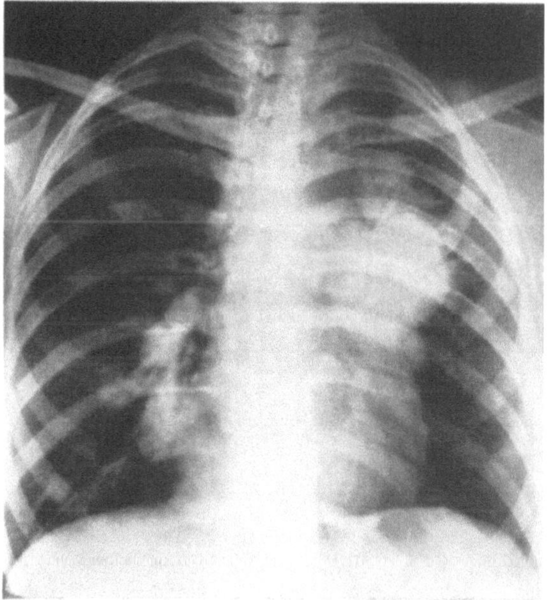

Fig. 27. Case B. B. Stage IV, 9. 2. 1967. Lung and mediastinal involvement. Ist. Oncologia-Torino

Tolerance is usually good. Administration may be oral or by intravenous injection, though the former may be accompanied by nausea and (rarely) gastric disturbances. Premedication with anticholinergics will control such disorders. Side effects are generally of little consequence and treatment can be continued (250 mg daily by intravenous injection, or oral maintenance doses, of 2—3×50 mg tablets per day) without interruption. Anorexia is the most likely complaint, but even vomiting and nausea should not be allowed to suspend treatment, except in rare instances. Alopecia is very rare (KENIS et al., 1965). Haematological damage is more evident though slow to appear. WBC and platelet values slowly fall, but not below critical levels; there is then a slow increase as a result of gradual adaptation. Other rare signs reported are: menstrual disturbances allergy dermatitis.

The results of treatment are considerable and include: gradual and constant improvement in subjective well-being, with reduction of fever, node enlargement,

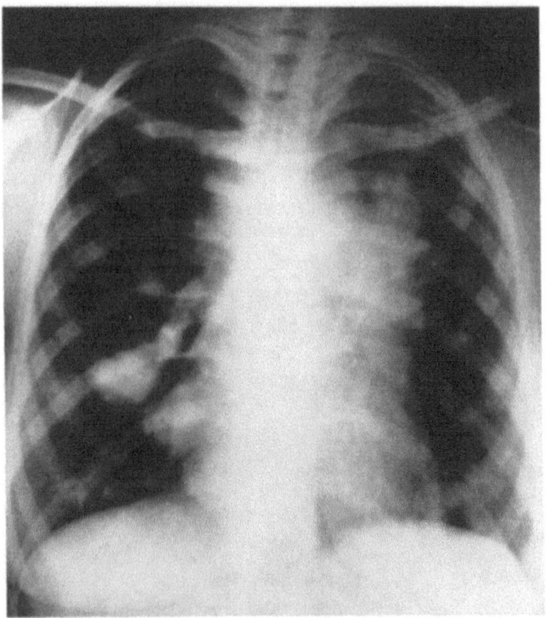

Fig. 28. Case B. B. Stage IV, 29. 3. 1967. Reduction of shadows in both fields during methyl-hydrazine treatment. Ist. Oncologia-Torino

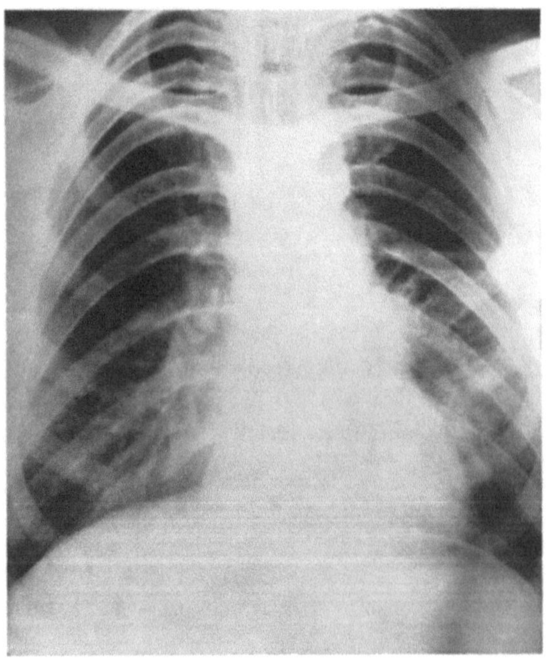

Fig. 29. Case B. B. Stage IV, 7. 5. 1967. Both fields cleared after methylhydrazine treatment. Ist. Oncologia-Torino

pruritus and pain, and regression of all general symptoms. These improvements appear slowly; decrease in spleen and liver enlargement is also slow. Cases of jaundice, with serious invasion of the epigastric region by (probably) tumoral masses, serious signs of toxicosis and very high serum bilirubin levels, have also been reported as showing progressive improvement: decrease and disappearance of infiltration, considerable sub-total decrease of liver size, normalisation of skin colour and other symptoms.

Remission is, however, of short duration (2—5 months); but normal conditions can be restored by repeated treatment. We have observed as many as 3 full cycles of complete remission following treatment with methylhydrazine. Our more recent practice is to continue maintenance therapy with oral doses of 100 mg per day. Cross-resistance is not observed and this drug can thus be used in cases that have resisted other forms of therapy.

4. Hormones

The antilymphatic and thymolytic properties of the corticosteroids are well known, even though the relationships between the position of lymphocytes in benign forms, the immunological status and steroid therapy are not fully understood. Steroid therapy undoubtedly has some effect on body defences and exercises, among many others, an anti-inflammatory activity which is the principal feature in this form of treatment.

Prednisone and prednisolone derivatives are most commonly used. Dosage varies from product to product though the effects are in each case much the same. High doses are employed in attack therapy (100—200 mg per day prednisolone; 40 to 50 mg per day triamcynolone; 7—10 mg per day dexamethazone; 5—10 mg per day betamethazone) whereas maintenance therapy uses correspondingly smaller doses (10—25 mg; 10—20 mg; 1—4 mg; 1—4 mg per day respectively).

Hormone therapy has a precise part to play in the management of Hodgkin's disease (FAUVET and ROUJEAU, 1960; GELLHORN, 1955); it should be called in as late and as little as possible (MOESCHLIN, 1960; STORTI et al., 1965). In one form, however, it is the treatment of choice: where the disease is persistently active and there is serious marrow lesion with leucopenia, radiotherapy is useless, fever and all general symptoms are fully in evidence and the disease is widespread. Steroid therapy is thus the only resource. Contraindications include: gastric ulcers, diabetes.

High (preferably oral) doses bring useful relief, with improvements in fever, lymph node size, and in general symptomatology. Remission is relatively rapid and may be maintained for weeks or months (DI GUGLIELMO et al., 1961; DUBOIS-FERRIÉRE, 1964). This may not be achieved if doses have to be reduced, but it is common for steroid therapy to bring the patient to a point where chemotherapy or even radiotherapy can be resumed. Where haemolytic anaemia is predominant, steroids are of great assistance.

The suggestion that high-dose steroid therapy should be used in every case of lymphomatous disease is not supported by facts (RANNEY and GELLHORN, 1957), though astonishing results are sometimes reported. Our practice is to use small doses for the maintenance therapy of subjects presenting only fever and malaise. In this way, a normal working life can be continued and radiotherapy or chemotherapy cycles can be spaced at longer intervals. An association of steroids and VLB sometimes produces good results and prevents further marrow damage. Side effects have already been noted, the most important being perforation of gastric ulcer. This can be avoided by obtaining prior knowledge of the condition and by suspension of treatment at the first sign of disturbance. Moon face, the reawakening of previous T. B. or the onset of osteoporosis lesions are harder to control and continuous check-ups are essential.

With respect to electrolyte status, blood sugar and B. P., steroids are today less dangerous, especially at low doses. If treatment is to be prolonged, however, salt intake should be reduced, a saluretic administered once or twice per week and potassium salts taken daily. Calcium loss may be countered with anabolising drugs, the risk of T. B. may be met by means of isonicotinic acid hydrazide and infection by the employment of antibiotics.

Steroids primarily depress tissue lymphocyte and eosinophile levels, whereas STERNBERG tissue is scarcely affected. Lymph nodes become softer and gradually decrease in size. Blood granulocyte levels rise in step with decreased lymphocyte values and there is enhanced serum protein production (KYLE, 1962).

5. Symptomatic Treatment

Other medical treatments are applied in the management of symptoms which resist the specific therapy being used; examples are fever, pain, pruritus, sweating, gastric disturbances etc.

Table 10. *Plan of treatments*

Treatment	Stages I and II	Stages III and IV	Maintenance
surgery	radical extirpation	palliative	
radiotherapy:			
— kilovoltages	200 r dose rate — total 2,000—3,000 r	local palliative	
— megavoltages	250 r dose rate — total 4,000—5,000 rads	local palliative	
nitrogen mustard	15—30 mg/1—5 days strategic forms	1.5—3 mg/day — total 30—50 mg	5 mg/every 2—3 *weeks*
TEM		2—4 mg/day — total 20—25 mg	
R 48		200—400 mg/day	
chlorambucil		10—20 mg/day — total 300 mg	
Thio-TEPA		10—15 mg/day — total 200 mg	10—15 mg/day
trisethyleneimino- benzoquinone		0.2—0.5 mg/day — total 4—8 gr	0.06 mg/day
cyclophosphamide		200 mg/day — total 3—7 gr	50—100 mg/day
vincaleucoblastine		10—15 mg/*week*	10 mg/*week*
methylhydrazine		250—300 mg/day	100 mg/day
prednisone		10—20 mg/day — total 40—80 (150—500 mg/day- massive)	5—10 mg/day

Fever may be the result of local infection or of the disease itself, including tissue necrosis, which is either a general feature of the disease or a sequela of radio- or chemotherapy (LOBELL et al., 1966). Phenylbutazone (HAMPEL et al., 1961), aminopyrine (SPEAR, 1962) and, more recently, indometacin (SILBERMAN et al., 1965; MARCOLONGO et al., 1966; PAVERO et al., 1966) have been used with success. These drugs enable periods of crisis to be overcome and specific treatment to be resumed. Apart from their anti-inflammatory action, these drugs appear to act directly on the CNS and can be used during the inter-cycle periods of chemotherapy.

Chapter III

Clinical Management of Hodgkin's Disease

In recent years a certain balance of opinion has been reached with respect to the management of the protean forms of this disease. The benefits of more modern forms of therapy are generally acknowledged and uniform treatment patterns have emerged. Results can be anticipated with greater certainty and prognosis is more accurate (KARNOFSKY et al., 1966). An important aspect of planned treatment is that damage is avoided and the patients' immunological status is unimpaired, since these factors are of essential importance in the determination of survival times.

1. Localised Forms (Stage I—II A)

As already pointed out, the course of the disease may be influenced very much from the earliness and quality of the initial treatment.

In Stage I cases, node mobility and depth must be carefully considered.

Many Centres now favour *radical excision of nodes* and this form of surgery has tended to replace biopsy. The operation will not always be easy nor are its results always predictable; the surgeon who sets out to perform a biopsy must, however, be prepared to proceed to more radical surgery designed to obtain a cure. In the words of PACK: "if biopsy were done more frequently and at the outset, the number of patients in unifocal Stage I could be increased and the possibility of radical operation enlarged". In his view, lasting success may be predicted in cases "where the disease is unifocal in form and presents a primarily nodular-sclerotic picture".

Contraindications to surgery include: 1. forms with widespread intestinal involvement (leaving aside primary gastro-intestinal forms); 2. PEL-EBSTEIN fever, or fever in general; 3. spleen enlargement; 4. generalized pruritus; 5. infection.

The operative field must be as wide as possible, so as to remove all regional foci and make subsequent radiotherapy unnecessary (SLAUGHTER, 1965; PACK et al., 1966). Results are rather good.

Surgery is clearly more suitable in young patients and in slow-moving forms with slight symptoms. Single-site primary gastro-intestinal forms are also amenable to surgical management.

Splenectomy, on the other hand, is not so readily recommended. Surgery does not give consistently good results (GRACE and MITTELMAN, 1966; PACK and MOLLANDER, 1966) and it is not always certain that the spleen is the only site.

Postoperative radiotherapy or chemotherapy is not universally practised. In our opinion, and in that of many workers, radiotherapy of the sites of immediate lymphatic drainage is an essential complement to surgery (PETERS, 1966). Others, e. g. SLAUGHTER, 1965, stress the "permanent and progressive" damage provoked by such therapy, whereas surgical cures are "stable". In some instances, surgery is suitable but contraindicated by e. g. skin damage following irradiation or lymph nodes firmly attached to deep tissue; here surgery involves unnecessary risk and is not advisable.

Radiotherapy (conventional, accelerators or cobalt techniques) is the other alternative in Stage I cases (KARNOFSKY, 1966), since "aggressive", high-dose treatment produces almost complete sterilisation of the disease site (RUBIN and KUROHARA, 1966). It is principally employed in forms localised in one or in a few sites, though all Stage I cases are suitable for such treatment, whether primary or recurrent (MUSSA, 1967). High-dose irradiation is suggested as the sole treatment in cases where surgery may spread the disease. Choice of treatment (surgery or radiation) will, however, depend on many factors (clinical picture, stage, etc.); the overriding need being to secure the complete extirpation of limited groups of diseased foci.

Some writers recommend chemotherapy as a complement to radiotherapy (MILLER et al., 1959). Survival times of 1—3 and 5 yrs have been obtained following the administration of NH_2 after main site and adjacent area irradiation doses of 2,500 rads and 1,000 rads respectively.

As a general rule, however, cytostatic treatment of localised forms is not recommended.

2. Regional Forms (Stages II—III A)

These are also regarded as localised forms and require obliterative irradiation, with or without the treatment of adjacent areas (GELLHORN, 1955). Complete remission lasting months or even years may be obtained.

Special localisations (mediastinum, spinal cord) (EASSON and RUSSEL, 1963) raise difficult questions of choice of treatment. Radiologists prefer cautious radiation management (BUSCHKE, 1965); chemotherapists suggest mixed forms of treatment with high initial doses of HN_2, to prevent the danger of radiation-induced congestion (GELLHORN, 1955; GRIFONI et al., 1965; GELLER, 1963).

Chemotherapy is also a useful alternative in cases of pulmonary hilar involvement, concomitant with mediastinal lesion, or in post-radiation recurrences. Where extensive pulmonary infiltration or skin damage are present, or a second or third course of X-ray treatment is requested, chemotherapy is clearly recommendable as an alternative to radiotherapy and a long course of HN_2 or one of the modern drugs will give equally good results (GELLER and LACHER, 1966).

Where the disease is localised in the abdomen, intensive radiotherapy can be delivered (FULLER, 1966) though in some cases it can aggravate such disturbances as diarrhoea, anaemia etc. and also lead to kidney complications. Chemotherapy is preferable, though here again renal function may be impaired.

Mediastinal forms with pleural effusion, though uncommon, are also classed as localised. Unilateral infiltration of the mediastinum may lead to stasis. Irradiation of the mediastinum, after pleural drainage, can be employed (KUZMA et al., 1966).

Peritoneal effusion is more rare and is the result of disseminated abdominal involvement or compression of hepatic veins following node enlargement (LENG-LÉVY et al., 1966); jaundice may also be present. For these cases, cautious chemotherapy is advised. Effusions may very occasionally be an expression of hypoproteinaemia and plasma or whole blood transfusion will be necessary. Repeated cycles of treatment with HN_2, thio-TEPA or cyclophosphamide are also of value.

3. Disseminated Forms

These form Stages III and IV, i. e. primary generalised forms, or recurrences following successful radiotherapy. In either case, *chemotherapy* is the treatment of choice, attention being given to the patient's general condition and drug-tolerance. HN_2 or, according to more modern methods, VLB is administered weekly, or methylhydrazine daily. We prefer to begin with methylhydrazine or VLB as they give marked improvement and general symptoms regression. VLB is advisable if gastric disturbances are present.

The choice of treatment will often be determined by previous experience and familiarity with one or other of the available substances. In any event, doses must be maintained at the selected level for long periods. While continuous haematological control is essential, falls in WBC to 3,000 or less are not a reason for suspension.

Our more recent experience indicates that remarkable, longlasting results can be obtained by alternating VLB and methylhydrazine; this method also helps to preserve the immunological status.

Enthusiastic recommendations in the literature in favour of different products are, of course, based on series of satisfactory responses (DE VITA et al., 1967). Stress must, however, be laid on the greater frequency of marrow toxicosis and side effects induced by cyclophosphamide, ethyleneiminobenzoquinone, mannitol mustard, etc. In the absence of special reasons, e. g. drug resistance, we prefer VLB or methylhydrazine for their comparative freedom from sequelae.

Oral administration of chlorambucil is still recommended by some writers, since this drug is of low toxicity and suitable for long-term use. While not denying its value, we would emphasize that its effects are slow to appear and depend on accumulation.

Steroid therapy is advisable in cases where prolonged cytostatic therapy has resulted in severe marrow damage. Clinical symptoms are improved and further damage is avoided. Such treatment may be combined with cytostatics but is more commonly practised alone. As STORTI, 1965, FAUVET et al., 1960, remarked, steroids should "put out the fire" rather than "break the back" of the disease. When the clinical signs have subsided to a certain extent, cytostatics, with or without radiotherapy, may be resumed. In cases where the patient's immunological defences have been impoverished by severe haematological lesions, fever and anaemia, and hope has been abandoned, steroid therapy may lead to the normalisation of general conditions. It is also recommended for primary (i. e. not treatment-induced) resistance, though it is more commonly employed in secondary cases.

Table 11. *Survival or remissions according to the various treatments*

Authors	Year	Case no.	Stage	Survival years			Remission			Observations
				3	5	10	c	n. c.	no	
				Radiotherapy						
Craver	1918—35	265	—		17.7%					
Craver	1930—43	471	—		23.6%					
Tubiana et al.	1922—48	46	I—II	36	19	2				
Tubiana et al.	1949—54	50	I—II	50	33	15				
Craver	1949—55	514	—		38.1%	9.9				
Roos and Videbaek	1930—45	172	—	52.3%	32.6%					
Hohl and Sarasin	1922—34	95	—		10.5%					
Hohl and Sarasin	1935—50	165	—		32.1%					
Nice and Stanstrom	1954	224	—		25	10				
Jeliffe and Thompson	1955	227	I—II—III		29					
Easson and Russel	1934—51	309	generalised	17.2%	11.02%					
Easson and Russel	1934—51	137	localised	56.0%	45.2%					
Kuentz	1955	170	—	42.0%	15.0%					
Hall et al.	1955	66	I—II—III	32.0%	24.0%					
Shimkin et al.	1955	254	I—II—III	44.6%	26.5%	7.6%				
Healy	1955	216	—		37	6				
Gellhorn et al.	1957	22	I	67.4%	36.8%					
Piemonte	1958				15.0%					
End result group	1950—57	458	M		23.0%					
End result group	1950—57	325	F		37.0%					
Peters	1960	285	I—II—III		36.1%	22.8%				
Hohl	1964	59	I—II—III	79.0%	62.8%					
Anaveri e Lucherini	1964	171	I—II—III		15.03%	5.26%				
Kaplan	1965	42	—		31.0%					2,000 v
Kaplan	1965	19	—		79.0%					4,000 v
Westling	1965	250	I—II	46.4%	35.6%	23.3%				
Heilmeyer et al.	1948—66	340	—		48.0%	28.7%				
Jeliffe	1966	298	I—II—III		30.0%	20.0%				

Table 11 (continued)

Authors	Year	Case no.	Stage	Survival years			Remission			Observations
				3	5	10	c	n. c.	no	
Lukes	1966	377	—		40.0%	22.0%				
Hancok	1967	45	—	71.6%	44.8%					
GECA-Radiobiology Group	1967	35	I—II A—B				68%			provisional data

Irradiation and chemotherapy

Authors	Year	Case no.	Stage	3	5	10	c	n. c.	no	Observations
Paterson	1954	256	—		25.0%					
Gellhorn et al.	1957	121	I—II—III	45.0%	25.7%					
Marchal et al.	1956	48	I—II—III	20	10					
Cook et al.	1922—57	347	—		34.6%					
Diamond	1958	713	I—II—III		17.1%	5.1%				
Paterson	1958	35	I		54.0%					
Anglesio	1952—66	85	II—III	56,0%	20.0%	10.0%				
Grifoni	1965	47	I—II—III		40.4%					
Di Pietro	1966	68	—		26.4%	5.8%				
Kuzma et al.	1966	58	II—III		29.3%					
GECA-Radiobiology Group	1967	37	I—II A—B				90% VLB			mediastinal provisional data

Chemotherapy

Authors	Year	Case no.	Stage	3	5	10	c	n. c.	no	Observations
unspecified										
Stacher	1966	146	III	33.6	13.3					
Nitrogen mustard										
Wilkinson	1955	80	I—II—III				78%		8%	
Larionov	1958	50	III	45.0%	25.7%					
Osgood	1958	31	III							
Karnofsky	1963	22	III		47.0%					

Table 11 (continued)

Authors	Year	Case no.	Stage	Survival years			Remission			Observations
				3	5	10	c	n. c.	no	
Chlorambucil										
GALTON	1955	23	III			4		14	5	
ULTMANN	1956	6	III			—		1	5	
BERNARD et al.	1957	52	—			17		25	20	
DE VRIES	1958	13	—			8		4	1	
ISRAELS	1958	35	III			11%		54%	35%	
ANGLESIO	1958	13	II—III			7		4	2	
Cyclophosphamide										
LASZLO	1962	11	III			45%				
GERHARTZ	1964	72	III			80%		30%	5%	
FAIRLEY	1966	62	—			69%			31%	
Trisethyleneiminoquinone										
LINKE	1960	134	III			96		21	17	
Vincaleucoblastine										
WHITELAW	1961	15	III			6		0	8	
WARWIK	1961	27	III					16	11	
HILL	1961	9	III			5		1	3	
KEISER	1962	22	III			3		4	2	
MATHÉ et al.	1962	9	III			7		9	6	
ARMSTRONG	1962	10	III			6		4		
OBRECHT	1964	20	III			5		1	3	
STUTZMAN	1966	33	III			15		5	3	
FAIRLEY	1966	62	—			18%			35%	
Methylhydrazine										
MARTZ	1964	25	—			25		25		
MATHÉ et al.	1964	51	III			17		5	3	
BRUNNER	1965	20	—			12		4	1	
WAGNER et al.	1965	12	—			7		28.0%		
HANSEN	1966	14	I—II—III			64.2%		2	8	
KENIS	1965	23	III			13		4	2	
ANGLESIO	1965	13	III			7		21	11	
WITTE	1966	44	—			12			19%	
SARTORIS et al.	1967	22	—			81%				

Alternation of treatment on resistant or untreated foci, associated with short radiation cycles will often lead to long periods of remission. Not only will the patient's own defences remain unimpaired, they can also be brought into play in the management of the disease, even in forms which appear to have reached the limits of every form of cure. Symptomatic treatment (transfusions, antibiotics, vitamins, etc.) are also important — (Table 11).

4. Treatment during Remissions

The problem of when and how to treat dormant forms or cases where clinical silence is almost complete is one of great importance. It is by no means uncommon to observe cases with scarcely palpable laterocervical nodes and no other signs; again, treated patients may be symptom-free and apparently normal on clinical examination.

Such cases must be kept under close observation and increased WBC or ESR should be taken as a sign for the recommencement of treatment. Similar considerations apply to cases presenting a small rosary of lymph nodes in the neck, with no other signs, or where low-grade fever or slight lymph node and or spleen enlargement indicate incipient recurrence.

The only time when treatment should be witheld is in cases that are completely silent, without signs of marrow damage.

A special group in this category consist of "benign" forms (DAWSON and HARRISON, 1961; WRIGHT, 1956, 1960). These are roughly equivalent to the histiocyte-lymphocyte forms or to paragranulomas. They must be kept under close observation and periodical check-up is essential. On the other hand, they may run a very long, clinically silent course and resist all attempts at cure.

Careful management during remission is never harmful; oral administration of chlorambucil, methylhydrazine, or weekly VLB enables the disease to be held for months, without limiting the use of other forms of treatment. Neglect, on the other hand, may well lead to recurrences and complications if remission has been only partial and these will be difficult to control. In all events, the extent of remission should not be overestimated and continuous check-up is essential.

Length of survival may well depend on accurate assessment of the histological picture and extent of disease (WESTLING, 1965). Forms with nodular sclerosis or lympho-histiocyte hyperplasia tend to run a protracted course with long symptom-free intervals and, for these, maintenance therapy with steroids may be the only advisable treatment. As soon as the clinical or radiological data indicate the onset of abnormalities, the patient's understandable tendency to let things slide must be contended with; more frequent check-ups must be carried out or a course of treatment set in motion.

5. Terminal Stages

Treatment is commonly abandoned in the terminal stage of all forms. Symptoms become ineluctable and disturbances unresponsive to continued radiation or drug therapy increase in number. Some writers (BERNARD, 1966; DUBOIS-FERRIÉRE, 1964; MOESCHLIN, 1960) have drawn attention to the fact that large doses of adrenocorticosteroids may be of assistance in such cases, or short massive courses of cyclo-phosphamide (STACHER, 1966).

300—400 mg of prednisone may be given for as long as 10—20 days under anti-biotic cover and dramatic improvement may follow (MOESCHLIN, 1960). Its duration is to be measured in weeks, though in some cases true remission may be obtained over a period of months and chemotherapy resumed. In the majority of patients, however, improvement will be limited to a temporary regression of symptoms, in particular fever and malaise.

6. Duration of Treatment

This is a controversial subject and is considered to be of paramount significance, though rarely discussed.

When lymph node size is again normal and clinical silence has been virtually achieved, there is a general tendency to suspend treatment so as to avoid further tissue damage. Experience shows, however, that, in the case of chemotherapy, maintenance doses should be administered for a further long period, under control in the case of radiotherapy; a total dose must be reached in any event.

It is generally considered that a firm therapeutic foundation must be established if inflammation and the other specific symptoms of Hodgkin's disease are to be completely suppressed. Rather than stop treatment, it is better to initiate maintenance therapy. In this way, good general condition may be preserved and an active life for months or even years is possible.

7. Resistance

One of the major problems faced by chemotherapists—though the radiotherapist is no stranger to it—is that of resistance. This may appear with any kind of drug and is usually a consequence of protracted treatment. On the other hand, the wide variety of products available make this problem less pressing, especially since the Vinca alkaloids and methylhydrazine do not give rise to cross-resistance.

The only way to avoid such a phenomenon is to interrupt the treatment and change to a different drug. Ethyleneimines, for instance, may be used in place of mustard derivatives or alkaloids. Steroid therapy can also be employed, as can colchicine on rare occasions.

8. General Disease Symptoms

The protean clinical forms of Hodgkin's disease mean that management must sometimes be extended to include symptoms of a more general character, when these are persistent or give rise to complications. It is not too much to say that there is no branch of medicine which may not be brought into the picture as a result of this disease. Some disturbances, therefore, may resist the specific therapy and require special (i. e. symptomatic) treatment.

Fever can be combatted with various drugs (e. g. antibiotics) if localised infection is suspected. Usually however, aspirin, pyrazolone, butazolidine, quinine or indo-metacin will be employed. Many writers recommend such substances as a form of subsidiary treatment, though the possibility of gastric disturbances or marrow toxicity must be kept in mind.

Pruritus is often refractory. Sometimes known as "Hodgkin's prurigo", this may be alleviated by cortisone, administered per os or locally (sprays or unguents).

Oral or hypodermic administration of phenothiazine derivatives may overcome resistant cases. Temporary benefit will be obtained by intravenous injection of novocaine or oral administration of procainamide. Hypnotic drugs can be given or Laborit mixture may be administered parenterally in saline solution.

Pain may sometimes require special treatment, especially at the outset of therapy, when effective dose levels have not yet been reached. Aspirin, pyrazolone derivatives, phenacetin and similar drugs give good results, but care must be taken to avoid marrow damage. More powerful drugs (e. g. opiates) are not often advisable. Associations of relaxant and analgesic drugs are frequently more effective.

Anaemia is commonly observed, especially in the advanced stages, and may sometimes be severe. Its management merits closer attention. Blood transfusions, together with the administration of iron preparations, are the normal means of treatment. In case of haemolytic anaemia, steroid therapy may give good results. Sometimes it is impossible to obtain improvement or to block haemolysis. Here, splenectomy is advised by some writers as a treatment for the secondary hypersplenism. If anaemia is the result of cachexia or loss, transfusions are mandatory.

Leucopenia may follow chemotherapy or be the expression of the effects of radiotherapy on bone marrow. In some advanced cases, it is a spontaneous manifestation of the disease. The treatment of choice is steroid therapy in association with transfusions. If WBC values are in the 3,000—4,000 range, antimitotic therapy may be cautiously continued. In the face of lower values, specific medical treatment will be essential. Hypersplenism-induced leucopenia may respond to cortisone or splenectomy.

Where primary leucopenia is present, cytostatics may induce a remission of the disturbances and an increase in white cell values (GELLHORN, 1955).

9. Special Forms

This term is to be taken as covering unusual sites or complications which disturb the course of the disease.

Dermatosis may present as a non-specific lesion (in 30⁰/o of cases, SAMMAN, 1966), accompanied by pruritus, or as a specific granulomatous lesion of the mycosis fungoides type. In the former case, cutaneous lesions such as deep pigmentation, particularly in dark-skinned subjects following intensive radiotherapy, may accompany pruritus; atrophy due to ichthyosis and exfoliative dermatitis affecting the whole body, particularly the face and eyes, are unusual rarities.

Some of these conditions may be handled with general chemotherapy and local improvement obtained. In the case of refractory forms, local application of steroid ointment is the only course open.

Herpes zoster is a well-known concomitant of Hodgkin's disease. Besides the commonest forms, varicelliform or extensive zoster-type eruptions with necrotic papulae may be observed (ERNER and SÖLTZ-SZÖTS, 1966; LEONARDI and MENOZZI,

1958; MAURO and PRATO, 1957; DAYAN et al., 1964; H. M. WILLIAMS et al., 1959). These are always an expression of deterioration, since they indicate further impairment of body defences (Fig. 30).

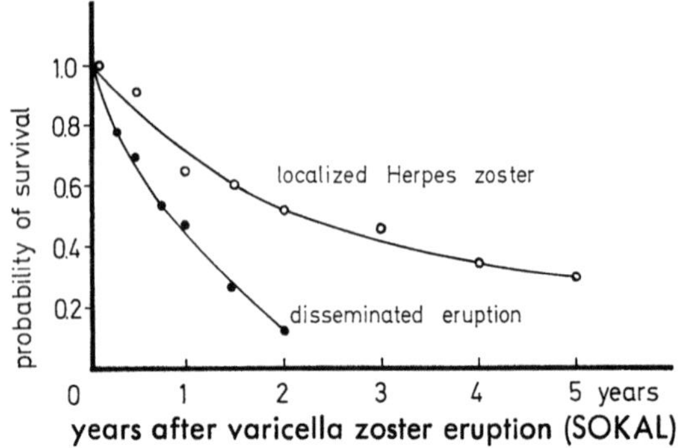

Fig. 30. Survival of patients after their first localized or disseminated varicella-zoster eruption (SOKAL)

Management of these forms requires great care; chemotherapy should be suspended so as to avoid further loss of immunological status and medical treatment should be restricted to the treatment of pain and fever. Many writers have referred to the conflict between the need to continue steroid therapy and that of avoiding further loss of immune defence (DAYAN et al., 1964). PINKEL considers gammaglobulin administration the best form of treatment.

Post-treatment remission of the disease itself may present herpes as the sole clinical sign and in such cases both local and general therapy will be directed to its cure.

The management of cutaneous lesions resulting from granulomatous infiltration or mycosis fungoides is more difficult (I. C. WRIGHT et al., 1960; SAMPEY, 1959; NAGY and MESZAROS, 1960). Necrosis and spontaneous ulceration readily follow such lesions and, although both radiotherapy and chemotherapy may bring improvement, the former may still favour further ulceration and treatment must be strictly supervised in every case.

Neurological forms include: 1. primary brain lesions, 2. spinal cord compression, 3. cranial nerve lesions, 4. peripheral nerve lesions, 5. multifocal disturbances.

Primary brain lesions are the least common (KAUFMAN, 1965). Symptoms are severe and include focal disturbances (paralysis, seizures, H. M. WILLIAMS et al., 1959) and signs of general involvement (confusion, coma) (HAYNAL and REGLI, 1964). Diffusion to the meninges as a result of contact or lesion of the skull is rare. Association of nitrogen mustard, steroids and, in some cases, radiotherapy may give temporary and, not infrequently, long-term improvement (STORTI, 1965; TODD, 1966; H. M. WILLIAMS et al., 1959).

Spinal cord compression presents symptoms that range from simple paraesthesia to complete paralysis and is attributable to infiltration of nerve roots via the intervertebral foramina, by epidural tumor diffusion from an adjacent vertebral site, or to ischaemia due to compression by granulomatous tissue.

The prognosis of Hodgkin's disease cases seems better than with other forms of lymphomas (H. M. WILLIAMS et al., 1959).

Treatment may take different forms. Early radiotherapy (conventional of megavoltage) gives good results and symptom regression may be dramatic. Its completeness will depend on the severity and the duration of the symptoms. Chemotherapy has been preferred since it first became available as a means of avoiding radiation-induced congestion (GELLHORN, 1955). Radiotherapy can then be resorted to, after large doses of cytostatics and a massive dose of steroids have been administered. In the case of less advanced lesions, medical treatment may be sufficient; in more severe cases, combined therapy is recommended, as also laminectomy.

Chemotherapy is also preferable in cases of peripheral nerve involvement, though lesion of the dura mater must be handled by radiation. In multifocal lesions, chemotherapy is clearly indicated.

Less frequently, neurological symptoms appear in the terminal or advanced stages as a consequence of steroids or chemotherapy. These include: brain abscess, meningeal reactions, multifocal leucoencephalopathy (KAUFMAN, 1965; HORWICH et al., 1951; TODD, 1966), i. e. lesions due to the subacute cerebellar degeneration, typical of the terminal picture of many neoplastic diseases and some reticuloses. Treatment meets with little response.

Bone involvement. The diagnosis of primary osteolytic or osteoplastic forms (more rare—TORRICELLI and CANOSSI, 1959) of Hodgkin's disease is complicated by the fact that these lesions simultate carcinoma metastases.

Surgical treatment is generally less successful than radiotherapy (conventional and megavoltage), though there are reports of total cure following eradication of the focus. Irradiation brings lasting improvement (PISANI and MALASPINA, 1957; MUSSHOFF et al., 1964) and almost complete repair; in a few cases, orthopaedic treatment may be required. In very rare cases, medical therapy must replace radiotherapy; in skull involvement, the underlying nervous tissue is threatened and irradiation must be taken with care.

Digestive apparatus. Localisation in the digestive apparatus is fairly common and requires particular attention.

The *oesophagus* is involved in 2 ways: by secondary infiltration from enlarged nodes or as a primary site (BICHEL, 1951; ENNUYER et al., 1961; STORTI et al., 1965; WEST and BOURONCLE, 1960). If the upper two-thirds are involved, an associated involvement of the cervical lymph nodes is common. In all forms, radiotherapy is the treatment of choice (CUCCIOLI, 1960). Improvement will include the relief of stenosis and may amount to a longlasting recurrence-free local cure.

There are many reported cases of *stomach* involvement (MARSHALL et al., 1959; MOUVET, 1960; McNEER and PACK, 1962; CORNES et al., 1966; KANE, 1963). This is almost always secondary and is a common feature of the terminal stages.

For primary forms, surgery gives good results (GREMMEL, 1958) and it is not uncommon for total or partial gastrectomy to be carried out because the lesion has been wrongly diagnosed as an epithelioma (KOLÁR and KÁCL, 1958; KANDOSHCHUK and KUCHERENKO, 1964).

Prognosis is good and the disease is often benign. Postoperative radiotherapy is a subject on which there is no general agreement. Such therapy is certainly to be recommended in secondary forms or where surgery is impracticable. Chemotherapy is also a suitable form of treatment in such cases.

Intestinal forms are also observed. The colon and ileum are the sites of choice, the other tracts being less frequently involved.

The difficulty of diagnosis means that primary forms are most often discovered intraoperatively (HOSKINS, 1966; COHEN and CANTER, 1959, RALSTON and WASDALL, 1958). Resection of the diseased segment and removal of the nodes may give long (GAMNA and PINO, 1939) or short (CORNES, 1966) periods of improvement, by comparison with the more hopeful prognosis of primary gastric forms (DAWSON et al., 1961). Excision is also recommended by COHEN and CANTER, 1959, especially in the case of the more severe symptoms presented by intestinal forms (TEITELMAN LLOYD and BRILL, 1960). This, in association with postoperative radiotherapy, can result in long survival times. On rare occasions, chemotherapy may be employed.

Pregnancy may raise difficult problems, touching both the course of the disease and that of gestation itself (GILBERT, 1961). Some authors advise Hodgkin's disease patients against marriage and, specifically, against childbearing (GELLHORN, 1955).

The course of pregnancy is uneventful during the remission period of a (usually benign) long-course form (HENNESSY and ROTTINO, 1963; GILBERT, 1961; HULTBERG, 1957; MINET, 1961; BONAZZI, 1958). Some years should elapse between an acute attack and the commencement of pregnancy. Some patients have had second pregnancy, with normal course and delivery, during remission phases; some have stated that they felt in excellent health during gestation (HULTBERG, 1957).

Spontaneous abortion (not always attributable to the disease) is observed in 7 to 10% of cases (VIRIEUX, 1966).

The course of the disease seems to be not different to that observed in non-pregnant patients (SMITH et al., 1958; BICHEL, 1950), though some distinction must be made (SCHULLER et al., 1966). As already stated, pregnancy occurring in a remission phase may well run to term without incident and be followed by normal delivery. On the other hand, exacerbation of the disease during pregnancy or post-partum may be observed (BARRY et al., 1962) and it is difficult to assess whether this is to be attributed to the natural course of the disease or to partus. Onset of the disease during pregnancy, or pregnancy occurring during an acute episode are much more serious and therapeutic abortion may have to be resorted to, although this has no effect on the disease itself (VIRIEUX, 1966).

If the disease is to be treated, close consideration must be given to the consequences for both mother and child (SMITH et al., 1958). In the majority of cases, treatment should be witheld. During remission periods, no changes of note take place and cases presenting slight symptom-free node enlargement can also be left untreated. Steroids should not be administered either, though there is no general agreement on this point. Radiotherapy must be localised and confined to extra-abdominal regions (or to the upper abdomen, if necessary); treatment should be delayed until late pregnancy, from the 6th month on, if possible, to avoid teratogenesis (GILBERT, 1961).

Obstetrical experience shows that no form of Hodgkin's disease is benefited by therapeutic abortion. This step should, therefore, only be undertaken in extremely severe cases, or when the onset of the disease falls in the first weeks of pregnancy. Every form requires energetic treatment at its first appearance and this is not always possible in the presence of pregnancy. Abortion will give the physician a freer hand. It should also be noted that a mutual negative influence between the disease and pregnancy is only found in cases where the initial onset occurs during gestation.

We may sum up by stating that, whereas every case should be most carefully investigated before proceeding, the general principle is that neither the pregnancy nor the disease will be affected by the association.

10. Complications

Infrequent, but dangerous, association of T.B. and Hodgkin's disease are known. Radiation, antimitotic and, in particular, steroid therapy may induce a loss of reactivity and depressed powers of resistance, which combine to trigger off a latent or unsuspected lesion. The incidence of T.B. diffusion as a direct cause of death is as low as 1—2%, however.

The presence of T.B. foci, especially in association with pulmonary lesions, must not be made the reason for suspending treatment. Complications due to the spread of infection can be contained by the association of anti-T.B. and radiation or anti-mitotic therapy. It is therefore advisable to proceed with the chosen treatment under antibiotic and anti-T.B. chemotherapeutic cover (STORTI et al., 1965; CRAVER, 1964).

Diabetes in Hodgkin's disease may be present in primary form (unsuspected by the patient) or as the result of steroid therapy. It may also be a concomitant condition which has already received treatment over a long period. It should, of course, be recalled that as steroid therapy is not a first line of attack, all treatments that do not cause further disturbances of sugar metabolism are to be preferred in most cases.

If severe diabetes is present, insulin can be associated with other forms of treatment. Steroid therapy, if essential, can be given for short periods, provided the metabolic picture is kept in balance with insulin or oral antidiabetics; the last are of greater use in less severe forms which have received no previous treatment.

Many *other complicating associations* may be met, which interfere with the carrying out of a proposed treatment plan. Except for the examples already dealt with, however, they rarely compel a radical change of programme or the suspension of therapy. Aggressive radiotherapy in Stage I or II cases may be obstructed by complications, though such interference is more likely to prevent the use of cytostatics or steroids. The presence of renal disturbances (nephrosis, amyloidosis) (STORTI et al., 1965), pericardial or myocardial infiltration, or the appearance of gastric or duodenal ulcers may be indications for the choice of a particular type of therapy, but are rarely the cause of serious restrictions on its execution.

Two more common occurrences, particularly in chronic cases, are: toxicosis, complicated by refractory haemolytic anaemia, and infection due to loss of immunological defence. The latter include: moniliasis, torulosis, cryptococcosis, toxoplasmosis (KEEL et al., 1963), aspergillosis, nocardiosis and mycormycosis (ULTMANN et al., 1966). These are not confined to the terminal stages and will obviously require individual treatment in each case.

Conclusions

On no other disease in the field of malignant tumours has the hand of change lain so heavily in the last 20 years as on Hodgkin's disease. Progress in pathology, the discovery of new drugs, the introduction of new forms of radiotherapy and the increased interest in surgical management have all played their part in the development of different forms of treatment and in the improvement of prognosis and of survival times (BERNARD, 1966).

Pathological studies, although as yet unable to supply a full account of the aetiopathogenesis of the disease, have introduced a new factor. Immunological behaviour studies have explained the significance of some components of lymphomatous tissue and prognosis is now reliably based on the incidence of such components in function of clinical stage and treatment received. This is an important fact in the interpretation of the improvements reported in the more recent literature.

New aids to diagnosis have made it possible to initiate suitable treatment at an earlier stage in several forms of the disease. An important example is lymphography, which can reveal every form of involvement, particularly of inaccessible nodes (retro-peritoneal, inguinal nodes). Stage classification is based on these findings and has contributed to improved assessment of treatment.

Renewed interest in surgical management has led to remarkable successes following radical excision in single-site forms; this is seen as confirmation of the fairly uniform diffusion of the disease.

The introduction of high-voltage radiotherapy has improved both results and management techniques. Decreased skin damage, the delivery of higher concentrations to deep foci and the larger doses employed have all contributed towards the many reported cases of success. Previously, indeed, radiotherapy appeared to have come to the end of its recources. In its rejuvenation, a large part has been played by the use of prophylactic or complementary therapy, i. e. the extension of irradiation to adjacent areas (PETERS, 1966; OSGOOD, 1958).

The most exciting developments, however, have been in the medical field. Nitrogen mustard had already revealed the potentialities of this form of treatment; and the discovery of new HN_2 derivatives, Vinca alkaloids and methylhydrazine has confirmed its promise. It may be claimed, in fact, that every stage of the disease is now able to be covered by a rational plan of treatment. Steroids, the universal panacea, have also been used to obtain both improvement and remission in forms once held to be past assistance. These various treatments can today be administered without reaching the level of marrow damage that was formerly a feature of unrestricted chemotherapy.

The combined experience of the many writers who have followed these developments over the years shows that a search must always be made for the most suitable of the three forms of therapy at present available. To adhere obstinately to the use of one such form only, without varying management in response to the course of the disease, is to ignore the progress that has been made, progress which has taken the survival figures to undreamed—of percentages and transformed Hodgkin's disease into one in which advances are continually being made.

To-day, prior agreement between surgeon, radiotherapist and chemotherapist is an essential prerequisite to the preparation of a plan of treatment, since the opinion of each of these specialists will eventually have to be sought in the majority of cases. Cooperation at the outset has been proved by the lessons of recent years to give the best advantages with the least risk of damage to the patient.

Future developments are hard to forecast. Even if no fresh aetiological evidence comes to light, immunology is likely to be the most promising field for new advances. A new, and not yet fully read, page has been opened by the interpretation of tissue features and their relationship to the behaviour of the disease. Skin tests and the study of serum proteins and blood cells may introduce new elements on which to base improved prognosis. Further research in this direction may lead to the addition of some new weapon to the already potent therapeutic armoury and to fresh advances in the field of immunotherapy.

References

AHMANN, D. L., J. M. KIELY, G. H. HARRISON, and W. S. PAYNE: Malignant lymphoma of the spleen. Cancer 19, 461 (1966).

AISENBERG, A. C.: Manifestations of immunologic unresponsiveness in Hodgkin's disease. Canc. Res. 26, 1152 (1966).

ANAVERI, G., e M. LUCHERINI: La malattia di Hodgkin. Nuntius Radiol. 12, 1323 (1964).

ANGLESIO, E.: Trattamento della malattia di Hodgkin con il Natulan. Min. med. 56, 4402 (1965).

— The treatment of systemic lymphomas with chlorambucil. Proc. VII. Congr. Intern. Soc. Haematology, Rome 1958.

—, A. CARBONARA, and G. MANCINI: Study of serum proteins in malignant lymphomas (in press).

ARENDS, T., C. V. CONRAD, and R. W. RUNDLES: Serum proteins in Hodgkin's disease and malignant lymphomas. Amer. J. Med. 16, 833 (1964).

ARMSTRONG, J. G., R. W. DYKE, P. J. FOUTS, and J. E. GAHIMER: Hodgkin's disease, carcinoma of the breast and other tumors treated with Vinblastine sulfate. Canc. Chem. Report 18, 49 (1962).

BACKHOUSE, T. W., and K. SICHER: Initial experiences with Methylhydrazine, a new cytotoxic agent. Clin. Rad. 17, 132 (1966).

BACQ, Z. M., and P. ALEXANDER: Fundamentals of radiobiology. 2nd Ed. Oxford: Pergamon Press 1961.

BARBIERI, D.: Quoted by FERRATA e STORTI.

BARRY, R. M., H. D. DIAMOND, and L. F. CRAVER: Influence of pregnancy on the course of Hodgkin's disease. Amer. J. Obst. Gyn. 84, 445 (1962).

BERNARD, J.: Principes généraux actuels du traitement de la maladie de Hodgkin, des lymphosarcomes, des réticuloses. Rev. Pract. 16, 871 (1966).

—, G. MATHÉ et M. WEIL: Traitement par l'acide P(di-2-chloro-éthylamino)phenilbutyrique de la maladie de Hodgkin, etc. Sang 28, 80 (1957).

BERNEIS, K., W. BOLLAG, M. KOFLER, and H. LUTHY: Synergismus between jonising radiation and a cytotoxic methylhydrazine derivative: effect on DNA-degradation. Experientia 21, 318 (1965).

Bichel, J.: Some investigations on the mechanism of the leukopenia produced by Vinca-leucoblastine. Acta path. micr. scand. 67, 1 (1966).
— Hodgkin's disease and pregnancy. Acta rad. 33, 427 (1950).
— Hodgkin's disease of the oesophagus. Acta rad. 35, 371 (1951).
Biesele, J. J.: Mitotic poisons and the cancer problem. Amsterdam: Elsevier 1958.
Bjerre Hansen, P., and J. Bichel: Triethylene melamine therapy in Hodgkin's and other malignant diseases. Acta rad. 35, 469 (1951).
Bollag, W.: The tumor-inhibitory effects of the methylhydrazine derivative Ro 4-6467/1. Cancer Chem. Report 33 (1963).
Bonazi, C. F.: Enfermedad de Hodgkin y embarazo. Prens. méd. Argent. 45, 2378 (1958).
Bond, W. H., R. J. Rohn, R. W. Dyke, and P. J. Fouts: Clinical use of triethylenemelamine. Report of 75 cases. Arch. int .Med. 91, 577 (1959).
Bostick, W. L.: Evidence for the virus etiology of Hodgkin's disease. Ann. N. Y. Acad. Sci. 73, 307 (1958).
Bousser, J.: Aspects cliniques de la maladie de Hodgkin et des sarcomes ganglionnaires. Rev. Pract. 16, 819 (1966).
Brunner, K. W., and C. W. Young: A methylhydrazine derivative in Hodgkin's disease and other malignant neoplasms. Ann. int. Med. 63, 69 (1965).
Bunting, C. H., and J. L. Yates: An etiologic study of Hodgkin's disease. J. Amer. med. Ass. 61, 1803 (1913).
Buschke, F.: Hodgkin's disease: Indication for radiation therapy. J. Amer. med. Ass. 191, 317 (1965).
Calciati, A., e M. Fazio: Intradermo-test con tubercolina deposito nel linfogranuloma maligno. Min. Med. 52, 3359 (1961).
Chase, M. W.: Delayed-type hypersensitivity and the immunology of Hodgkin's disease, with a parallel examination of sarcoidosis. Canc. Res. 26, 1097 (1966).
Chevallier, P., et G. Bilski-Pasquier: Maladie de Hodgkin ou Lymphgranulomatose maligne Traité de Médecine. Paris: Masson & Cie 1949.
Chiappa, S.: La radioterapia endolinfatica nel trattamento delle linforeticolopatie sistemiche. J. Belge Radiol. 47, 657 (1964).
—, G. Bonadonna, C. Uslenghi, G. Galli, P. Marano, and A. Molinari: Current views and recent results on endolymphatic radiotherapy in the treatment of malignant lymphomas. (In press).
Cohen, N., and J. W. Canter: Hodgkin's disease of the small intestine: report of six cases. Amer. J. Digest Dis. 4, 361 (1959).
Congdon, Ch. C.: The destructive effect of radiation on lymphatic tissue. Canc. Res. 26, 1211 (1966).
Cook, J. C., K. L. Krabbenhoft, and T. Leucutia: Combined radiation and nitrogen mustard therapy in Hodgkins' disease as compared with radiation therapy alone. Amer. J. Roentgen. 82, 651 (1959).
Cornes, J. S.: Hodgkin's disease of the gastro-intestinal tract. Proc. roy. Soc. Med. 60, 732 (1966).
Craver, L. F.: Recent advances in treatment of lymphomas, leukemias and allied disorders. Bull. N. Y. Acad. Med. 24, 3 (1948).
— Treatment of Hodgkin's disease. Treament of cancer and allied diseases. New York: Harper and Row 1964.
Croizat, P., et R. Creyssel: Les troubles des protéines du sérum dans les hémopathies malignes. Rev. Pract. 11, 587 (1961).
—, P. Galy, J. Papillon, L. Revol, J. L. Chassard et G. Bretagnolle: Les formes média-stinales de debut de la maladie de Hodgkin. J. Radiol. 43, 1 (1942).
Cuccioli, U.: Su di una localizzazione primitiva esofagea del linfogranuloma maligno. Arch. ital. Mal. Appar. dig. 27, 150 (1960).
D'Alessandri, A., H. J. Keel, W. Bollag u. G. Martz: Erste klinische Erfahrungen mit einem neuen Cytostaticum. Schweiz. med. Wschr. 93, 1018 (1963).
Dameshek, W., L. Weissfuse, and T. Stein: Nitrogen mustard therapy in Hodgkin's disease: analysis of 50 consecutive cases. Blood 4, 338 (1949).

DAWSON, I. M. P., I. S. CORNES, and B. C. MORSON: Primary malignant lymphoid tumors of the intestinal tract. Brit. J. Surg. **49**, 80 (1961).

DAWSON, P. S., and C. V. HARRISON: A clinicopathological study of benign Hodgkin's disease. J. clin. Path. **14**, 219 (1961).

DAYAN, A. D., H. G. MORGAN, H. F. HOPE-STONE, and B. J. BOUCHER: Disseminated Herpes Zoster in the reticuloses. Amer. J. Roentg. **92**, 116 (1964).

DEL VECCHIO, S., e C. SANDOMENICO: La terapia radiante del linfogranuloma maligno. Rev. Radiol. **6**, 1191 (1966).

DE VITA, V. T., and A. SERPICK: Combination chemotherapy in the treatment of advanced Hodgkin's disease. Proc. Amer. Ass. Canc. Res. **8**, 49 (1967).

DEVOIS, A., et R. DECKER: L'avenir de la maladie de Hodgkin traitée. Sem. Hôp. **30**, 197 (1954).

DE VRIES, S. I.: Treatment of malignant lymphomas with chlorambucyl. Acta haemat. **19**, 1 (1958).

DIAMOND, H. D.: Results of therapy in Hodgkin's disease. Ann. N. Y. Acad. Sci. **73**, 357 (1958).

DI GUGLIELMO, R., A. MILIANI, V. LOMBARDI, F. ZINI e A. ZILLI: Effect clinici e umorali indotti dalla terapia con prednisone a dosi elevate in alcune emopatie e altre situazioni morbose. Haemat. **46**, 309 (1961).

DI PIETRO, S.: Risultati a distanza di 100 casi di malattia di Hodgkin trattati con chemoterapia. Tumori **53**, 111 (1967).

—, e L. V. GIACOMELLI: Le ipriti azotate e la chemioterapia dei tumori maligni. Tumori **40** (1954).

—, e C. USLENGHI: Primi risultati della radioterapie endolinfatica nel linfogranuloma maligno. Tumori **51**, 113 (1965).

—, e F. PIZZETTI: La prognosi istologica del granuloma maligno in base allo studio di 100 casi. Tumori **52**, 451 (1966).

DUBIN, I. N.: Poverty of immunological mechanism in patients with Hodgkin's disease. Ann. int. Med. **27**, 898 (1947).

DUBOIS-FERRIÈRE, H.: Le traitement actuel des leucémies aigues et des lymphomes malins en stade de généralization. Méd. Hyg. (Genève) **16**, 464 (1964).

EASSON, E. C.: Possibilities for the cure of Hodgkin's disease. Cancer **19**, 345 (1966).

—, and M. H. RUSSELL: The cure of Hodgkin's disease. Brit. med. J. i, 1704 (1963).

EBNER, H., u. J. SÖLTZ-SZÖTS: Generalisierter Herpes Zoster bei Morbus Hodgkin. Zschr. Haut- u. Geschl.-Kr. **41**, 85 (1966).

End Result Group: Mortality trends in cancer. N. C. I. monography n. 6 (1961).

ENNUYER, A., P. BATAINI et J. HÈLARY: Maladie de Hodgkin des voies aéro-digestives supérieures. Ann. Oto-laryng. **78**, 474 (1961).

ESTEVEZ, R. A.: Use of mannitol derivative of nitrogen mustard. Sem. Med. **125**, 281 (1964).

FAIRLEY, G. H., M. J. L. PASTERSON, and R. B. SCOTT: Chemotherapy of Hodgkin's disease with cyclophosphamide, vinblastine and procarbazine. Brit. med. J. ii, 75 (1966).

FAUVET, J., et J. ROUJEAU: Les dérivés cortisoniques dans le traitement du cancer et de la lymphogranulomatose maligne. Rev. Pract. **10**, 2405 (1960).

FAZIO, M., P. CAVALLERO, S. SARTORIS, F. VERGNANA e L. PEGAROLO: Prime esperienze cliniche con metilidrazina nel trattamento del linfogranuloma maligno. Min. Med. **56**, 99 (1965).

FELCI, U.: Terapia radiologica dei tumori linforeticolari. Atti Soc. It. Cancerologia, Milano 1967.

FERRATA, A., e E. STORTI: Le malattie del sangue. Milano: Vallardi 1958.

FORBUS, W. D., and J. U. GUNTER: Pathogenicity of strains of brucella obtained from case of Hodgkin's disease. South. med. J. **34**, 376 (1941).

FLURY, R., u. T. WEGMANN: Das Verhalten der alkalischen Leukocytenphosphatase beim morbus Hodgkin. Schweiz. med. Wschr. **94**, 958 (1961).

FULLER, L. M.: Results of large volume irradiation in the management of Hodgkin's disease and malignant lymphomas originating in the abdomen. Radiology **87**, 1058 (1966).

—, and G. H. FLECHTER: The radiotherapeutic management of the lymphomatous diseases. Amer. J. Roentg. **88**, 909 (1962).

FULLER, L. M., B. JING, C. C. SCHULLENBERGER, and J. J. BUTLER: Radiotherapeutic management of Hodgkin's disease involving the mediastinum. Proc. roy. Soc. Med. 60, 730 (1966).

GALL, E. A.: The surgical treatment of malignant lymphoma. Ann. Surg. 118, 1064 (1966).

GALTON, D. A. G., L. G. ISRAELS, J. D. M. NABARRO, and A. M. TILL: Clinical trials of P(di-2-chlorethylamino)phenylbutiric acid (C. B. 1348) in malignant lymphomas. Brit. med. J. ii, 1172 (1955) .

—, M. TILL, and E. WILTSHAW: Busulfan (1,4-dimethansulfonoxibutane)Myleran. Summary of clinical results. Ann. N. Y. Acad. Sci. 68, 967 (1958).

GAMNA, C., e F. PIINO: Il linfogranuloma maligno gastro-intestinale. Arch. ital. Mal. Apper. dig. 8, 312 (1939).

GARY-BOBO, J.: Premiers résultats des traitements par la Vincaleucoblastine des maladies de système et des sarcomes (association à la radiothérapie). Antitumoral effects of Vinca Rosea Alkaloids. Amsterdam: Excerpta Medica Found. 1966.

GELLER, W.: The mandate for chemotherapeutic decompression in superior vena caval obstruction. Radiol. 81, 387 (1963).

—, and M. J. LACHER: Hodgkin's disease. Med. Clin. N. Amer. 50, 819 (1966).

GELLHORN, A.: Management of the patients with Hodgkin's disease. J. chron. Dis. 1, 698 (1955).

— End results in lymphosarcoma and Hodgkin's disease. Proc. 3rd Nat. Canc. Conf. Philadelphia: Lippincott 1957.

—, and V. P. COLLINS: A quantitative evaluation of the contribution of nitrogen mustard to the therapeutic management of Hodgkin's disease. Ann. int. Med. 35, 1250 (1951).

GERHARTZ, H.: Clinical results with cyclophosphamide and trisethylene iminoquinone. In: PLATTNER: Chemotherapy of cancer. Amsterdam: Elsevier 1964.

GILBERT, R.: The problem of pregnancy in Hodgkin's disease. Acta radiol. 35, 71 (1961).

GOLDMAN, I. M., and I. R. HOBBS: The immunoglobulins in Hodgkin's disease. Immunology 13, 421 (1967).

GOODMAN, L. S., M. M. WINTROBE, W. DAMESHEK, M. J. GOODMAN, A. GILMAN, and M. T. McLENNAN: Nitrogen mustard therapy. Use of methyl-bis(β-chloroethyl)-amine hydrochloride and tris (β-chloroethyl)-amine hydrochloride for Hodgkin's disease, lymphosarcoma, leukemia and certain allied and miscellaneous disorders. J. Amer. med. Ass. 132, 126 (1946).

GOULIAN, M., and J. L. FAHEY: Abnormalities in serum proteins and protein bound exose in Hodgkin's disease. J. Lab. clin. Med. 57, 408 (1961).

GRACE, J. T., and A. MITTELMAN: Surgery in the management of Hodgkin's disease. Cancer 19, 351 (1966).

GREMMEL, H.: Die primäre Lymphogranulomatose des Magens. Die Med. 24, 977 (1958).

GRIFONI, V., S. TOGNELLA, G. BIGNOTTI, A. FORNI, G. GASPARINI e C. CONFALONIERI: Stato attuale della terapia della malattia di Hodgkin. Rec. Prog. Med. 39, 585 (1965).

GROLLMAN, A., R. L. JOHNSON, and W. W. REGAN: A clinical evaluation of colchicine in the treatment of Hodgkin's disease. Ann. int. Med. 42, 154 (1955).

GROSS, R., u. K. LAMBERS: Erste Erfahrungen in der Behandlung maligner Tumoren mit einem neuen N-Lost-Phosphamidester. Dtsch. med. Wschr. 83, 458 (1958).

HALL, C. A., and K. B. OLSON: Prognosis of the malignant lymphomas. Ann. int. Med. 44, 687 (1956).

HAMMER, B: Ergebnisse radiologisch-zytostatischer Kombinationsbehandlung maligner Erkrankungen. Wien. med. Wschr. 117, 637 (1967).

— Zur Behandlung des Lymphogranuloms. Wien. med. Wschr. 116, 562 (1966).

HAMPEL, K. E., D. ALGENSTAEDT u. H. GERHATZ: Zur Butazolidinbehandlung menschlicher Hämoblastosen. Blut 7, 398 (1961).

HAN, T., and L. STUTZMAN: Mode of spread in patients with localized malignant lymphoma. Arch. int. Med. 120, 1 (1967).

HANCOCK, P. E. T., and E. M. LEDLIE: Treatment of early Hodgkin's disease. Lancet i, 26 (1967).

HANSEN, M. M., H. HERTZ, and A. VIDEBAEK: Use of a methylhydrazine derivative especially in Hodgkin's disease. Acta med. scand. 180, 211 (1966).

HANSON, T. A. S.: Histological classification and survival in Hodgkin's disease. Cancer 17, 1595 (1964).

HARE, H. F., B. M. DAHLE, and J. G. TRUMP: Two million-volt X-ray therapy of Hodgkin's disease. Ann. N. Y. Acad. Sc. 73, 363 (1958).

HARDER, J.: Über Knochenlymphogranulomatose. Fortschr. Röntgenstr. 93, 445 (1960).

HEYNAL, A., u. F. REGLI: Neurologische Symptome bei Morbus Hodgkin. Schweiz. med. Wschr. 94, 1515 (1964).

HEALY, R. J., H. I. ARNERY, and M. FRIEDMAN: Hodgkin's disease: a review of two hundred and sixteen cases. Radiology 64, 51 (1955).

HEILMEYER, L., u. K. MUSSHOFF: Die Therapie der Lymphogranulomatose und die Frage ihrer Heilbarkeit. Münch. med. Wschr. 109, 2109 (1967).

HENNESSY, J. P., and A. ROTTINO: Hodgkin's disease in pregnancy. Amer. J. Obst. Gyn. 87, 851 (1963).

HILL, J. M., and E. LOEB: Treatment of leukemia, lymphoma and other malignant neoplasms with vinblastine. Canc. Chemother. Rep. 15, 41 (1961).

HODGKIN, TH.: One some morbid appearances of the absorbent glands and spleen. Medico-Chir. Trans. 17, 68 (1832).

HOFFBRAND, B. I.: Hodgkin's disease and hypogammaglobulinemia, a rare association. Brit. med. J. i, 1156 (1964).

HOHL, K.: Heutiger Stand der Therapie und Prognose der Lymphogranulomatose. Radiol. Clin. 33, 273 (1964).

—, PH. SARASIN u. W. BESSLER: Therapie und Prognose der Lymphogranulomatose. Oncologia 4, 1 (1951).

HORWICH, L., P. H. BUXTON, and M. S. RYAN: Cerebellar degeneration with Hodgkin's disease. J. Neurol. Neurosurg. Psychiat. 29, 45 (1951).

HOSKINS, E. O. L.: Unusual radiological manifestations of Hodgkin's disease. Proc. roy. Soc. Med. 60, 729 (1966).

HULTBERG, S.: Pregnancy in Hodgkin's disease. Acta radiol. 41, 277 (1957).

ISRAELS, L. G., D. GALTON, M. TILL, and E. WILSHAW: Clinical evaluation of CB 1348 in malignant lymphoma and related diseases. Ann. N. Y. Acad. Sci. 68, 915 (1958).

JACKSON, A.: Primary Hodgkin's disease of the stomach. Amer. J. Surg. 94, 546 (1957).

JACKSON, F. C., E. G. NEY, and E. R. FISHER: Surgical implantation of Hodgkin's disease of the stomach to the skin of the abdominal wall. Ann. Surg. 150, 1000 (1959).

JACKSON, H., and F. PARKER: Hodgkin's disease and allied disorders. New York: Oxford Univ. Press 1947.

JACOBSON, L. O., C. L. SPURR, E. S. GUZMAN BORRON, T. SMITH, C. LUSHBOUGH, and G. F. DICK: Nitrogen mustard therapy. Studies on the effect of methyl-bis(β-chloroethyl)amine hydrochloride on neoplastic disease and allied disorders of the hemopoietic system. J. Amer. med. Ass. 132, 263 (1946).

JELIFFE, A. M.: Facteurs influant sur la survie à long terme des malades atteints de maladie de Hodgkin. Nouv. Rev. franç. Haemat. 7, 85 (1966).

— Factors in early cancer which influence the prognosis: Hodgkin's disease. Proc. roy. Soc. Med. 59, 605 (1966).

—, and A. D. THOMPSON: The prognosis in Hodgkin's disease. Brit. J. Cancer 9, 21 (1955).

KANDOSHCHUK, T. A., and A. E. KUCHERENKO: Diagnostic difficulties in localized Hodgkin's disease of the gastrointestinal tract. Klin. Chir. 4, 9 (1964).

KANE, A. A.: Hodgkin's disease of the stomach. Amer. J. Gastroent. 40, 504 (1963).

KAPLAN, H. S.: The radical radiotherapy of regionally localised Hodgkin's disease. Radiology 78, 553 (1962).

— Evidence of a tumoricidal dose level in the radiotherapy of Hodgkin's disease. Canc. Res. 26, 1221 (1966).

— Role of intensive radiotherapy in the management of Hodgkin's disease. Cancer 19, 356 (1966).

— Clinical evaluation and radiotherapic management of Hodgkin's disease and malignant lymphomas. New Engl. J. Med. 278, 892 (1968).

KARNOFSKY, D. A.: The staging of Hodgkin's disease. Canc. Res. 26, 1090 (1966).

— Chemotherapy of Hodgkin's disease. Cancer 19, 371 (1966).

KARNOFSKY, D. A.: Hodgkin's disease: Chemotherapy. J. Amer. med. Ass. **191**, 30 (1965).

—, J. K. BURCHENAL, G. C. ARMSTEAD, C. M. SOUTHAM, J. L. BERNSTEIN, L. F. CRAVER, and C. P. RHOADS: Triethylene melamine in the treatment of neoplastic disease. Arch. int. Med. **87**, 477 (1951).

—, D. G. MILLER, and R. F. PHILLIPS: Role of chemotherapy in the management of early Hodgkin's disease. Amer. J. Roentgenol. **90**, 968 (1963).

KAUFMAN, G.: Hodgkin's disease involving central nervous system. Arch. Neur. **13**, 555 (1965).

KEEL, H. J., W. ROTH, G. KEISER, F. REUER u. G. MARTZ: Über das Zusammentreffen von Morbus Hodgkin' und Toxoplasmose. Schweiz. med. Wschr. **93**, 1465 (1963).

KEISER, G., K. BRUNNER u. G. MARTZ: Klinische Erfahrungen mit VLB (Velbé) einem neuem Cytostaticum. Schweiz. med. Wschr. **92**, 486 (1962).

KENIS, Y.: Etude comparée de la Vincaleucoblastine et du Natulan dans la maladie de Hodgkin. Antitumoral effects of Vinca Rosea Alkaloids. Amsterdam: Excerpta Medica Found 1966.

—, J. WERLI, J. H. HILDEBRAND et H. J. TAGNON: Action d'un dérivé de la methylhydrazine, le Ro 4.6467, dans la maladie de Hodgkin, dans d'autres lymphomes malins et dans les leucémies. Europ. J. Cancer **1**, 33 (1965).

KOLÁR, J., u. J. KÁCL: Zur Diagnostik von malignen Lymphomen des Magen-Darm-Kanals. Med. Klin. **53**, 140 (1958).

KOPP, H., u. R. HEINEKER: Zur Behandlung von bösartigen Lymphknotentumoren mit Cyclophosphamid. Dtsch. med. Wschr. **90**, 1257 (1965).

KRUMBHAAR, E. B.: The presetn status of Hodgkin's disease. Symposium on the blood and blood-forming organs. Wisconsin Univ. press: Madison 1939.

KUENTZ, M.: Etude statistique, clinique et thérapeutique de la granulomatose maligne. A propos de 170 observ. Thèse de Lyon 1955.

KUMMER, H., u. U. BUCHER: Erfahrungen mit einem neuen Zytostaticum der Methylhydrazinreihe (Natulan.) Schweiz. Med. Wschr. **95**, 31, 1233 (1965).

KUNDRAT, H.: Ueber Lympho-sarkomatosis. Wien. klin. Wschr. **6**, 211 (1893).

KUZMA, I., J. JANČINA, and J. ĎURKOWSKY: Therapeutic results in mediastinal localization of lymphogranulomatosis. Neoplasma **13**, 185 (1966).

KYLE, R. A., C. E. McPARLAND, and W. DAMESHEK: Large doses of prednisone and prednisolone in treatment of malignant lymphoproliferative disorders. Ann. int. Med. **57**, 717 (1962).

LACHER, M. J.: Role of surgery in Hodgkin's disease. New Engl. J. Med. **268**, 289 (1963).

LANE, M., B. LIPOWSKA, TH. C. HALL, and J. CALSKY: A preliminary report: observations on the clinical pharmacology of 5[bis(2-chloroethyl)amino](uracil mustard: MSC 34 462). Canc. Chemother. Report **9**, 31 (1960).

LARIONOV, L. F.: Immediate and remote results of chloroethylamine treatment of Hodgkin's disease. Brit. med. J. **i**, 252 (1956).

LASZLO, J., J. GRIZZL, U. JONSSON, and R. W. RUNDLES: Comparative study of mannitol mustard, cyclophosphamide and nitrogen mustard in malignant lymphomas. Canc. Chemother. Report **16**, 247 (1962).

LEE, B. J.: Lymphangiography in Hodgkin's disease: indications and controindications. Canc. Res. **26**, 1084 (1966).

LENG-LÉVY, J., J. DAVID-CHAUSSÉ, B. LENG, P. MAGENDIE et M. BELLET: Les formes coelomiques de la maladie de Hodgkin. J. Méd. Bordeaux **143**, 1727 (1966).

LEONARDI, P., e L. MENOZZI: Sul valore semeiologico e clinico dello Zoster nelle emoblastosi. Acta med. patav. **18**, 185 (1958).

LETTRÉ, H.: Action of vincaleucoblastine upon cells in vitro and against Ehrlich ascites tumours. Antitumoral effects of Vinca Rosea Alkaloids. Excerpta Med. Found.: Amsterdam 1966.

LEVITT, W. M.: Large-volume radiotherapy. Brit. J. Radiol. **28**, 75 (1955).

LINKE, A.: Die Behandlung der Haemoblastosen und der bösartigen Geschwülste mit Trisethylen Iminobenzokinon. Dtsch. med. Wschr. **85**, 1928 (1960).

LOBELL, M., D. R. BOGGS, and M. M. WINTROBE: The clinical significance of fever in Hodgkin's disease. Arch. int. Med. **117**, 335 (1966).

Longcope, W. T., and K. R. McAlpin: Hodgkin's disease. Oxford Med. 4, part. 1 (1920).

Longo, P., e V. Beltrami: Linfogranuloma di Hodgkin a localizzazione principale splenica. (Possibilità e limiti della splenectomia.) Ann. Fac. Med. Chir. Perugia 49, 179 (1958).

Lukes, R. J.: Relationship of histologic features to clinical stages in Hodgkin's disease. Amer. J. Roentgenol. 90, 944 (1963).

— Prognosis and relationship of histologic features to clinical stages. J. Amer. med. Ass. 190, 914 (1966).

Maggiorelli, L., G. Faleg e A. Pazzagli: Patologia del granuloma maligno nei vari distretti del canale alimentare. Arch. De Vecchi 30, 147 (1959).

Magrassi, F.: Quoted by Ferrata e Storti.

Marchal, G., L. Mallet et G. Duhamel: Traitement de la maladie de Hodgkin. Paris: Doin & Cie. 1956.

Marcolongo, R., e C. A. Boggiano: Sull'azione antipiretica della'indometacin nel linfogranuloma di Hodgkin e nelle neoplasie. Min. Med. 57, 2857 (1966).

Marmont, A., e F. A. Fusco: Una nuova sostanza antiblastica, la vincaleucoblastina nel trattamento delle emolinfoblastosi. La Clin. Ter. 25, 301 (1964).

Marsden, J. A.: Report on the use of vincaleucoblastine in the cases of Hodgkin's disease. Med. J. Austr. 2, 100 (1963).

—, and E. E. Damasio: Studies on the effects of two alkaloids from Vinca Rosea on human malignant cells in vivo. I. The effects of vinblastine in Hodgkin's disease. Proc. 10th Congr. Europ. Soc. Haematology, Strasburg 1965.

Marshall, S. F., and N. E. Adamson: Sarcoma of the stomach. Surg. Clin. North Amer. 39, 711 (1959).

Martz, G., A. D'Alessandri, J. Keel, and W. Bollag: Preliminary clinical results with a new antitumor agent, Ro 4-6467. Canc. Chemother. Report 33, 5 (1963).

Mathé, G., L. Berumen, O. Schweissguth, M. Schneider, J. L. Amiel, A. Cattan, L. Schwarzenberg et G. Brulé: Essai de traitement par une méthylhydrazine de la maladie de Hodgkin et de divers hématosarcomes et leucémies. Presse méd. 72, 1641 (1964).

—, M. Schneider, P. Bond, J. L. Amiel, L. Schwarzenberg, A. Cattan et J. R. Schlumberger: Leurosine sulfate (NSC 90 636) in treatment of Hodgkin's disease, acute lymphoblastic leukemia and lymphoblastic lymphosarcoma. Canc. Chemother. Report 49, 47 (1965).

—, O. Schweissguth, G. Brulé, J. L. Amiel, A. Cattan, M. Thomas et P. Zamet: Essai de traitement de la maladie de Hodgkin et d'autres affections réticulohystiocytaires malignes par la Vincaleucoblastine. Presse méd. 70, 1349 (1962).

Mauro, G., e V. Prato: L'herpes zoster nelle leucemie e nel linfogranuloma. Min. Med. 48, 2954 (1957).

McNeer, G., and G. T. Pack: Malignant tumors of the stomach. In: Pack and Ariel: Treatment of cancer and allied diseases. New York: Hober 1962.

Melli, G., e V. Grifoni: Terapia delle emoblastosi. Atti 61° Cong. Medicina Interna, Napoli 1960.

Miller, D. G., H. D. Diamond, and L. F. Craver: The clinical use of chlorambucil. A critical study. New Engl. J. Med. 261, 525 (1959).

Minet, P.: Grossesse et lymphogranulomatose maligne. Etude de sept cas d'association. Presse méd. 69, 1617 (1961).

Moeschlin, S.: Langzeitbehandlung der Hämoblastosen. Dtsch. med. J. 17, 551 (1960).

Monahan, D. T.: Hodgkin's disease of the lung. J. thorac. cardiovasc. Surg. 49, 172 (1965).

Mouvet, W.: Les localisations gastriques des „lymphomes malins". J. Belge Radiol. 43, 553 (1960).

Mussa, L.: Il trattamento radiante del morbo di Hodgkin. Giorn. Accad. Med. Torino 130, 294 (1967).

Musshoff, K., M. Busch u. H. Kaminski: Lymphogranulomatose (Morbus Hodgkin) mit Knochenbefall etc. Fortschr. Röntgenstr. 101, 117 (1964).

Nagy, E., and K. Meszaros: Experiences with Degranol in the treatment of mycosis fungoides. Magyar. Onkol. 4, 57 (1960).

Nice, C. N., and K. W. Stenstrom: Irradiation therapy in Hodgkin's disease. Radiol. 62, 641 (1954).

OBRECHT, P., G. MÖSSNER, H. STRICKSTROCK u. W. J. WOENCKHAUS: Die Therapie der Lymphogranulomatose und des Retikulosarcoms mit dem Zytostaticum Velbe. Beitr. Inn. Med. Stuttgart: Schattauer 1964.

—, K. H. STRICKSTROCK u. H. WEIBLEDER: Klinische und lymphographische Verlaufskontrolle bei Lymphogranulomatose und Retothelsarcom unter Behandlung mit Natulan. Europ. J. Cancer 2, 59 (1966).

OSGOOD, E. E.: Methods of analysing survival data illustrated by Hodgkin's disease. Amer. J. Med. 24, 40 (1958).

PACK, G. T., and D. W. MOLANDER: The surgical treatment of Hodgkin's disease. Canc. Res. 26, 1254 (1966).

PAGLIARDI, E., and E. GIANGRANDI: Clinical significance of the blood copper in Hodgkin's disease. Acta haemat. 24, 201 (1960).

PALTAUF, R.: Lymphosarcom. Ergebn. allgem. Path. path. Anat. 3, 652 (1896).

PAPILLON, J., P. CROIZAT, L. REVOL, J. L. CHASSARD, J. FEROLDI, A. CONTAMIN et L. DUTON: Les survies de plus de 10 ans dans la maladie de Hodgkin. Nouv. Rev. franç. Haem. 6, 79 (1966).

— — — —, F. BOTHIER et J. COSTE: Les localisations osseuses de la lymphogranulomatose maligne. J. Radiol. Électrol. 45, 109 (1964).

PARSONS, P. B., and M. A. POSTON: Pathology of human brucellosis; report of four cases with one autopsy. South. Med. J. 32, 7 (1939).

PATERSON, E.: Evaluation of chemotherapeutic compounds in the reticuloses. Brit. J. Cancer 12, 332 (1958).

—, P. B. KUNKLER, and A. L. WALPOLE: Triethylenemelamine in human malignant disease: results with oral administration of enteric-coated tablets. Brit. med. J. i, 59 (1953).

PAVERO, A., e S. DELLA PIETRA: L'impiego dell'indometacin nel trattamento della febbre nella linfogranulomatosi maligna. Arch. Maragl. 22, 541 (1966).

PETERS, M. V.: Hodgkin's disease: radiation therapy. J. Amer. med. Ass. 191, 28 (1965).

— Prophylactic treatment of adjacent areas in Hodgkin's disease. Canc. Res. 26, 1232 (1966).

—, T. C. BROWN, J. W. DAVIDSON, V. S. SAXENA, and M. SAINI: The value of locating occult disease in the treatment of Hodgkin's disease. Progress in Lymphology. Stuttgart: Thieme 1967.

—, and K. CH. MIDDLEMISS: A study of Hodgkin's disease treated by irradiation. Amer. J. Roentgenol. 79, 114 (1956).

PIEMONTE, M.: Considerazioni terapeutiche sul linfogranuloma maligno. Lezioni sui tumori. Vol. IV, Udine 1965.

PINKEL: Quoted by Storti.

PISANI, G., e A. MALASPINA: Le localizzazioni scheletriche del linfogranuloma maligno. Min. Med. 48, 2213 (1957).

RALSTON, L. S., and W. A. WASDALL: Gastrointestinal Hodgkin's disease. Amer. J. Gastroent. 29, 537 (1958).

RAMIOUL, H.: Les differents aspects cliniques et radiologiques des localisations pulmonaires de la maladie de Hodgkin. Acta Clin. Belg. 15, 1 (1960).

RANNEY, H. M., and A. GELLHORN: Effect of massive prednisone and prednisolone therapy on acute leukemia and malignant lymphomas. Amer. J. Med. 22, 405 (1957).

RATTI, A.: La radioterapia endolinfatica con I^{131}. Primi risultati. Rad. Clin. 31, 220 (1962).

REED, D. M.: On the pathological changes in Hodgkin's disease with special references to its relation to tuberculosis. Johns Hopkins Hosp. Rep. 10, 133 (1902).

RIGAT, L.: Rendiconto clinico-statistico dei linfoblastomi maligni trattati del 1928 al 1949. II. Il linfogranuloma maligno. Rad. Med. 44, 438 (1958).

ROOS, D., and A. VIDEBAEK: Prognosis in Hodgkin's disease. Dan. med. Bull. 6, 177 (1959).

ROSENBERG, S. A., and H. S. KAPLAN: Evidence for an orderly progression in the spread of Hodgkin's disease. Canc. Res. 26, 1225 (1966).

ROTTINO, A.: Therapeutic results in treatment of Hodgkin's disease with CB 1348 and R 48. Blood 12, 755 (1957).

— Triethylene melamine in treatment of Hodgkin's disease and other lymphomas. N. Y. St. J. Med. 52, 346 (1952).

ROTTINO, A., and A. LEVY: Behaviour of total serum complement in Hodgkin's disease and other malignant lymphomas. Blood **14**, 246 (1959).

ROUSSELOT, L. M., A. J. RELLA, and A. ROTTINO: Splenectomy for hypersplenism in Hodgkin's disease. Amer. J. Surg. **103**, 769 (1962).

RUBIN, P.: Hodgkin's disease. J. Amer. med. Ass. **190**, 910 (1964).

— Hodgkin's disease. Comment: pregnancy and childhood. J. Amer. med. Ass. **191**, 318 (1965).

—, and S. S. KUROHARA: Has prophilactic irradiation proved itself in the treatment of localised Hodgkin's disease? Radiol. **87**, 240 (1966).

RUNDLES, R. W., E. V. CONRAD, and N. L. WILLARD: Summary of results obtained with TEM. Ann. N. Y. Acad. Sci. **68**, 926 (1958).

SAMMAN, .P D.: Hodgkin's disease: Cutaneous manifestations. Proc. roy. Soc. Med. **60**, 736 (1966).

SAMPEY, J. R.: Chemotherapeutic management of mycosis fungoides. A survey of 224 cases. Amer. J. Pharm. **131**, 152 (1959).

SARTORIS, S., C. BACHI, D. BLEFARI, P. CAVALLERO, F. VERGNANO e N. FAZIO: La metilidrazina nel trattamento del morbo di Hodgkin. Min. Med. **59**, 296 (1968).

SCHAMAUN, M.: Chirurgische Behandlungsmöglichkeiten der Lymphogranulomatose. Praxis **55**, 754 (1966).

— Surgical treatment of Hodgkin's disease. Progress in Lymphology. Stuttgart: Thieme 1967.

SCHIER, W. W.: Cutaneous anergy and Hodgkin's disease. New Engl. J. Med. **250**, 353 (1954).

SCHULLER, L., I. COJOLAN, I. LÖRINCZ, S. OLARIN, and T. SHAPIRA: Primary malignant lymphogranulomatosis of the stomach associated with pregnancy. Oncologia (Basel) **20**, 291 (1966).

SCHWARZ, G.: The role of lymphangiography. Hodgkin's disease. J. Amer. med. Ass. **190**, 912 (1964).

SCOTT, R. M., and M. E. BRIZEL: Time-dose relationships in Hodgkin's disease. Radiology **82**, 1043 (1964).

SELLEI, C., and S. ECKHARDT: Clinical observations with 1,6 bis(beta chloroethylamino)-1,6-deoxy-D-mannitol dihydrochloride (BCM) in malignant diseases. Ann. N. Y. Acad. Sci. **68**, 1164 (1958).

SHIMKIN, M. B.: Hodgkin's disease: Effectiveness of treatment in control. J. Amer. med. Ass. **190**, 916 (1964).

—, K. C. OPPERMANN, W. L. BOSTICK, and B. V. A. LOW-BEER: Hodgkin's disease: an analysis of frequency, distribution and mortality at the University of California Hospital 1914—1951. Ann. int. Med. **42**, 137 (1955).

SICHER, K., and T. W. BACKHOUSE: Experiences with methylhydrazine. Brit. med. J. **i**, 858 (1965).

SILBERMAN, H. R., T. G. MacGINN, and W. B. KREMER: Control of fever in Hodgkin's disease by indometacin. J. Amer. med. Ass. **194**, 597 (1965).

SILVERBERG, J. H., and W. DAMESHEK: Use of triethylenemelamine in treatment of leukemia and leukosarcoma. J. Amer. med. Ass. **148**, 1015 (1952).

SLAUGHTER, D. P.: Hodgkin's disease: radical surgery. J. Amer. med. Ass. **191**, 26 (1965)

—, S. G. ECONOMOU, and H. W. SOUTHWICK: Surgical management of Hodgkin's disease. Ann. Surg. **148**, 705 (1958).

SMETANA, H. F., and B. M. COHEN: Mortality in relation to histologic type in Hodgkin's disease. Blood **11**, 211 (1956).

SMITH, D. F., and C. T. KLOPP: The value of surgical removal of localised lymphomas. Surg. **49**, 469 (1961).

SMITH, R. S. W., TH. W. SHEEY, and H. ROTHBERG: Hodgkin's disease and pregnancy. Case report and discussion of the treatment of Hodgkin's disease and leukemia during pregnancy. Arch. int. Med. **102**, 777 (1958).

SOKAL, J. E.: Immunologic unresponsiveness in Hodgkin's disease. Canc. Res. **26**, 1161 (1966).

SPEAR, W.: The use of aminopyrine to control fever in Hodgkin's disease. J. Amer. med. Ass. **180**, 148 (1962).

Stacher, A.: Ergebnisse der zytostatischen Therapie maligner Hämatoblastosen. Wien. Z. inn. Med. **47**, 1 (1966).

Sternberg, C.: Ueber eine eigenartige unter dem Bilde der Pseudoleukämie verlaufende Tuberkulose des lymphatischen Apparates. Z. Heilk. **19**, 21 (1898).

Stolberg, H. D., N. L. Patt, K. F. MacEven, O. H. Warwick, and T. C. Brown: Hodgkin's disease of the lung: roentgenologic-pathologic correlation. Amer. J. Roentgenol. **92**, 96 (1964).

Storti, E.: Peut-on considérer la lymphogranulomatose comme une maladie à debut localisé? Necessité d'un diagnostic précis. Soc. Med. Paris 754 (1937).

—, e S. Perugini: La terapia del linfogranuloma maligno nella pratica. Arch. Med. Mutual. **44** (1965).

Stramignoni, A., V. Canino e F. Mollo: Aspetti morfologici della malattia di Hodgkin con riferimento alla prognosi. Giorn. Accad. Med. Torino **130**, 259 (1967).

Stutzman, L., E. Z. Ezdiuli, and M. A. Stutzman: Vinblastine sulfate versus cyclophosphamide in the therapy for lymphoma. J. Amer. med. Ass. **195**, 173 (1966).

Svoboda, G. H.: Current status of research on the alkaloids of vinca rosea linn. Antitumoral effect of Vinca Rosea alkaloids. Amsterdam: Excerpta Med. Found. 1966.

Syke, P. et al.: Quoted by Marchal.

Teitelman, Lloyd S., and N. R. Brill: Localised Hodgkin's disease of the small intestine. Amer. J. Surg. **69**, 247 (1960).

Todd, I. D. H.: Intracranial lesions in Hodgkin's disease. Proc. roy. Soc. Med. **60**, 734 (1966).

Todd, D. M.: A methylhydrazine derivative (Ro 4-6467) in the management of late Hodgkin's disease and other lymphoreticular neoplasms. Brit. Med. J. **i**, 628 (1965).

Torricelli, A., e G. Canossi: Considerazioni su di un caso di linfogranuloma maligno con localizzazioni osteosclerotiche al rachide (vertebra d'avorio) e al bacino. Ann. Radiol. Diagn. **32**, 1 (1959).

Trousseau: Quoted by Chevallier et Bilski-Pasquier.

Tubiana, M.: Tendences nouvelles dans la radiothérapie de la maladie de Hodgkin. Oncologia 20, suppl. 4 (1966).

—, A. J. Laugier, M. J. Schlienger et G. Juillard: La radiotherapie de la maladie de Hodgkin. Rev. Pract. **16**, 911 (1966).

— —, M. Hayat, E. Attie et G. Mathé: Essai d'association radiotherapie-chimiothérapie dans le traitement de la maladie de Hodgkin. Nouv. Rev. Franç. Hémat. **6**, 134 (1966).

Uehlinger, E.: Über Knochenlymphogranulomatose. Virch. Arch. **288**, 36 (1933).

Ultmann, J. E.: Chemioterapia del linfoma. Aggiorn. Emat. **3**, 203 (1966).

—, J. K. Cunningham, and A. Gellhorn: The clinical picture of Hodgkin's disease. Canc. Res. **26**, 1047 (1966).

—, G. A. Hyman, Ch. Crandall, H. Naujoks, and A. Gellhorn: Triethylenethiophosphoramide (Thio-TEPA) in the treatment of neoplastic disease. Cancer **10**, 903 (1957).

— —, and A. Gellhorn: Chlorambucil in treatment of chronic lymphocytic leukemia and certain lymphomas. J. Amer. med. Ass. **162**, 178 (1956).

Vaitkevicius, V. K., R. W. Talley, J. L. Tucker, and M. J. Brennan: Cytological and clinical observations during vincaleucoblastine therapy of disseminated cancer. Cancer **15**, 294 (1962).

Virieux, C.: Evolution de la maladie de Hodgkin associée à une grossesse. Rev. Méd Suisse Rom. **86**, 821 (1966).

Wagner, K., H. Haas u. A. Meyerhold: Erfahrungen mit Natulan. Behandlung von Lymphogranulomatosen und Retikulosarcomatosen. Wien. klin. Wschr. **36**, 589 (1965).

Wagner, O.: Die Eosinophilie und das Hautjucken bei Lymphogranulomatose. Schweiz. med. Wschr. **78**, 745 (1948).

Warwick, O. H., R. E. Alison, and J. M. Darte: Clinical experience with vinblastine sulfate. Canad. med. Ass. J. **85**, 579 (1961).

Weitzel, G., F. Schneider u. A. M. Fretzdorff: Cytostatischer Wirkungsmechanismus der Methylhydrazine. Experientia **20**, 38 (1964).

West, W. O., and B. A. Bouroncle: Spontaneous perforation of the oesophagus in Hodgkin's disease. Report of three cases and literature review. Amer. J. Gastroent. **33**, 335 (1960).

WESTLING, P.: Studies on the prognosis in Hodgkin's disease. Acta radiol. Suppl. 245, (1965).

WHITELAW, D. M., and J. M. TEASDALE: Vincaleucoblastine in the treatment of malignant disease. Canad. med. Ass. J. 85, 584 (1961).

WILLIAMS, H. M., H. D. DIAMOND, L. F. CRAVER, and H. PARSONS: Neurological complications of lymphomas and leukemias. Springfield, Ill.: Thomas 1959.

WILLIAMS, R. D., N. C. ANDEWS, and R. P. ZANES: Major surgery in Hodgkin's disease. Surg. Gyn. Obst. 93, 636 (1951).

WILKINSON, J. F.: The chemotherapeutic treatment of the reticuloses. Proc. roy. Soc. Med. 48, 365 (1955).

—, M. S. BOURNE, and M. C. G. ISRAELS: Treatment of leukemias and reticulosis with uracil mustard. Brit. med. J. i, 1563 (1963).

WILKS, S.: Cases of enlargement of the lymphatic glands and spleen. Guy's Hosp. Report 11, 56 (1865).

WISE, N. B., and M. A. POSTON: Coexistence of brucella infection and Hodgkin's disease. J. Amer. med. Ass. 115, 1976 (1940).

WITTE, S., H. MARTIN u. J. C. F. SCHUBERT: Über die cytostatische Therapie mit einem Methylhydrazinderivat. Schweiz. med. Wschr. 96, 93 (1966).

— u. K. TH. SCHRICKER: Die zytostatische Therapie der Lymphogranulomatose. In Therapie maligner Tumoren, Hämoblastome und Hämoblastosen, Bd. I, Pathologie and Chemotherapie. Stuttgart: Enke 1966.

WRIGHT, C. I. E.: Hodgkin's paragranuloma. Cancer 9, 773 (1956).

— The "benign" form of Hodgkin's disease (Hodgkin's paragranuloma). J. Path. Bact. 80, 157 (1960).

WRIGHT, J. C., S. L. GUMPERT, and F. M. COLOMB: Remission produced with the use of Methothrexate in patients with mycosis fungoides. Canc. Chemotherap. Report 9, 11 (1960).

ZELLER, P., H. GUTMANN, B. HEGEDÜS, A. KEISER, A. LANGEMANN, and M. MÜLLER: Methylhydrazine derivatives, a new class of cytotoxic agents. Experientia 19, 129 (1963).

ZIEGLER, .K: Die Hodgkinsche Krankheit. Jena: Fischer 1911.

ZOGRAPHOV, D. G.: Ein Beitrag zur Kasuistik der Lymphogranulomatose. Akute Lymphogranulomatose. Zschr. inn. Med. 16, 565 (1961).

Author Index

Subject Index

Herstellung: Konrad Triltsch, Graphischer Betrieb, Würzburg

MIX
Papier aus verantwortungsvollen Quellen
Paper from responsible sources
FSC® C105338

If you have any concerns about our products,
you can contact us on
ProductSafety@springernature.com

In case Publisher is established outside the EU,
the EU authorized representative is:
Springer Nature Customer Service Center GmbH
Europaplatz 3, 69115 Heidelberg, Germany

Printed by Libri Plureos GmbH
in Hamburg, Germany